Heal Your Leaky Gut Diet and Meal Plan

Heal Your Leaky Gut Diet and Meal Plan

The Natural Detox Program to Improve Digestive Health

David Brownstein, MD
with Jodie Gould

To the women of my life: Allison, Drs. Hailey and Jessica, with all my love.

To physicians not satisfied with the dogma, who are willing to search for a new paradigm that promotes health.

And to all those who believe that the human body has a remarkable capacity to be healthy if given the proper raw materials.

CONTENTS

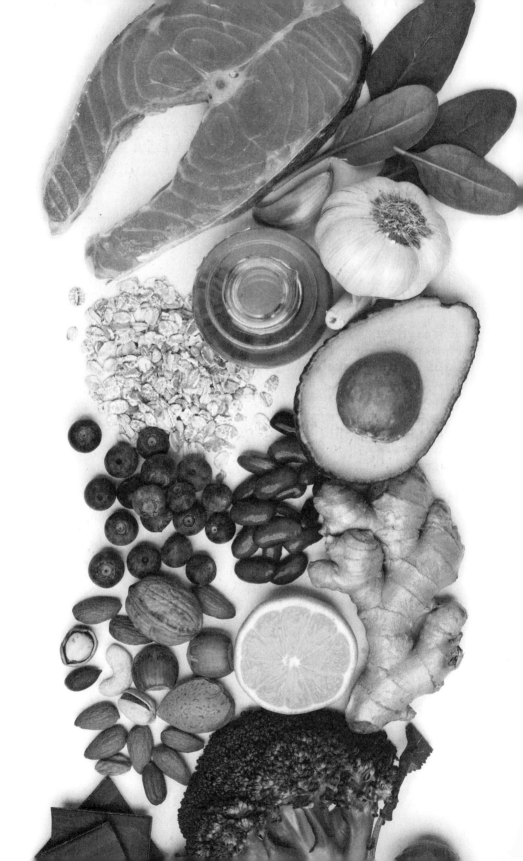

Introduction

Ever since I was a young boy, I wanted to be a family doctor. I came from a traditional Jewish household where physicians were revered, their advice never questioned. I held on to this belief through medical school, where we were given a lone, three-hour course on nutrition because it was not considered a priority in our training. I learned how to diagnose illnesses and treat them with medications. We were taught that supplements didn't work and that using them was like setting fire to your money.

After completing my residency, I opened a family practice in a Detroit, Michigan, suburb. Six months into what I thought was my life's calling, I told my wife that I no longer wanted to be a doctor. I was almost 30 and deep in student debt; we were about to welcome our first child. My wife, Allison, did not take the news well, but she could see how painfully unhappy I was and knew that I could not continue. We had no idea how we would support a family if I left medicine.

After many sleepless nights, I was introduced by a colleague to Dr. Robert Rade, a chiropractor who was also an expert in nutrition. At the time, I didn't trust the chiropractic profession, but I decided in my sleep-deprived haze to meet with him nonetheless. He told me about an entirely different way to treat patients using vitamins, minerals, herbs, and alternative therapies. He also gave me a book called *Healing with Nutrition* by Jonathon Wright, MD, an allopathic practitioner, which I read that night.

From that moment on, I vowed to learn as much as I could about nutrition and to study holistic medicine, which treats the whole person rather than just the symptoms of a disease. I discovered that natural therapies—and how we nourish our bodies—are the keys to good health. Today, after nearly 30 years as medical director at the Center for Holistic Medicine in West Bloomfield, Michigan, I have successfully treated thousands of patients for a variety of ailments and chronic diseases. I learned that many of these conditions stem from problems in the gut. Chief among them is leaky gut syndrome (LGS), which affects millions of people, many of whom are unaware they have it.

This was the case for Angela*, a 33-year-old registered nurse who came to me with stomach pains. She suffered from bouts of diarrhea, constipation, and bloating. I was the third doctor she had consulted. Both her previous physicians had diagnosed her with irritable bowel syndrome (IBS) without ever discussing her diet, even though she asked them if her stomach issues were caused by something she ate. Both also prescribed medications, none of which worked.

When I saw Angela, I gave her a physical exam and took a complete medical and dietary history. I discovered that her diet

The name has been changed in the interest of privacy.

was loaded with dairy, including lots of cheese, and refined carbohydrates such as bread and pasta. Her lab tests revealed a high level of antibodies to the cow's milk protein called casein (pronounced KAY-sin). Antibodies are a protein produced by the body's immune system when it detects a harmful substance. This did not surprise me because a majority of the people I see are allergic to casein. She also tested positive for *H. pylori*, a bacterial infection of the stomach lining.

I told Angela to immediately switch to a dairy-free diet. I also treated her with an herbal therapy consisting of oregano oil, Citricidal® (made from grapefruit rind), and mastic, an herb from the Mediterranean that peer-reviewed studies have shown to be effective in treating *H. pylori*. When I saw her again eight weeks later, she was fully recovered.

The good news is that, like Angela, you are able to heal if you supply your body with the basic raw materials it needs to optimally function. You might think LGS impacts only the digestive system. But as I wrote in *Heal Your Leaky Gut*, LGS can lead to numerous conditions, including IBS, allergies, arthritis, depression, anxiety, eczema, lupus, multiple sclerosis, type 1 diabetes, and chronic fatigue. I estimate that 80 percent of people with chronic illnesses have leaky gut, which affects the gut lining. (For a complete explanation of LGS, see Chapter 1.)

Changing what you eat and drink is one of the best strategies for getting your body back on a healthy track. In this book, I outline the steps you can take to change your diet: what to shop for, how to organize your pantry, how to stay motivated, and what lifestyle tips will help you heal. By eliminating "Gut Guzzlers" (the foods and beverages that make you sick) and replacing them with "Good Gut" foods, herbs, and nutrients, you will feel better and have more energy. As a bonus, you might even get leaner if you're carrying some extra pounds. I will also explain the brain-gut connection and hormonal factors that are important to maintaining gut health. Your journey back to health through proper nutrition can happen in just eight weeks!

The delicious and easy-to-make recipes in this book were created by Sheryl Shenefeld, a certified nutritionist who has co-authored many of my other food-related books. The recommended meals, desserts, and snacks have all been carefully curated to avoid processed foods loaded with additives or foods ordered from a drive-through window. Ideally, our foods should be as close to their natural state as possible and come from locally sourced, non-factory farms. The food on this meal plan will not only taste good, but they won't leave you feeling deprived or hungry in order to get healthy!

In the back of this book is a symptom tracker and a food diary where you can record your meals and your progress. I invite you to visit me at drbrownstein.com, sign up for my blog updates, and let me know how your symptoms improve over the coming weeks. Good luck on your journey to health.

To all our health!

David Brownstein, MD

PART 1

What to Eat for A Healthy Gut

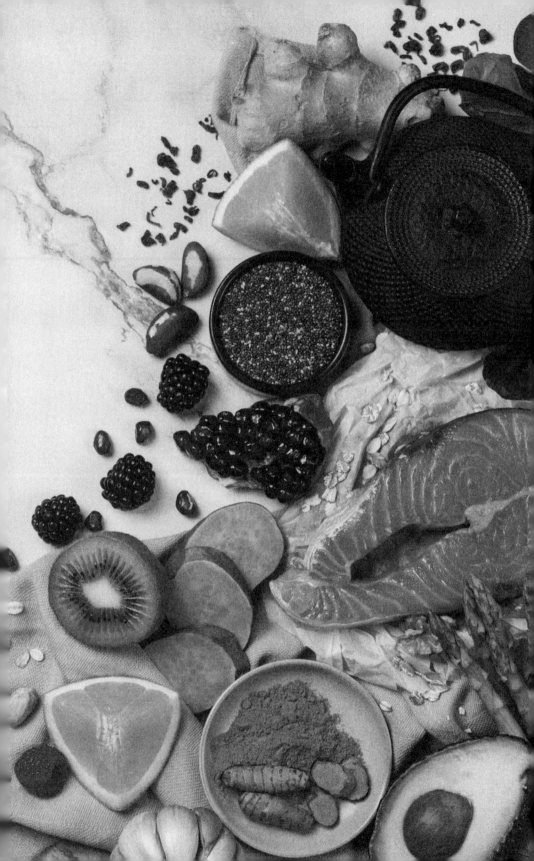

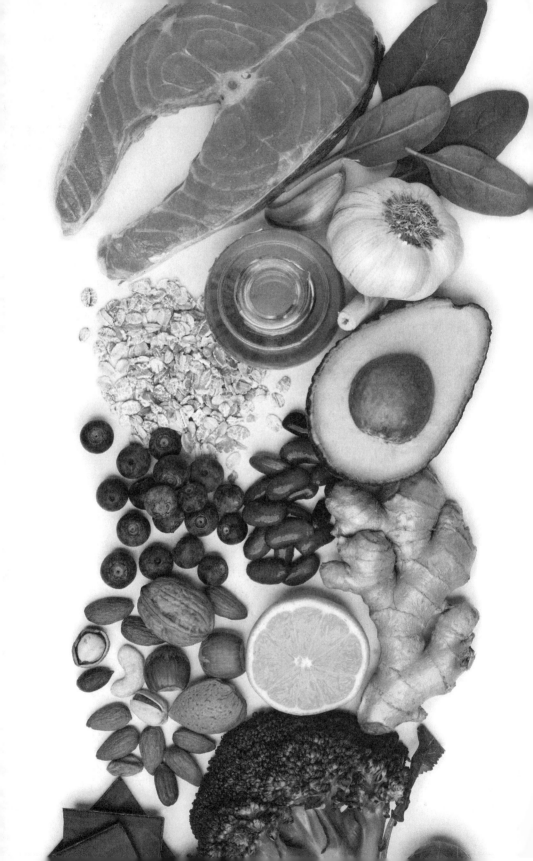

CHAPTER 1

What Is Leaky Gut Syndrome (LGS)?

Before I explain what LGS is, let's start with a brief biology lesson. The gut is another name for the gastrointestinal (GI) tract that includes the organs of the digestive system. During digestion, nutrients are extracted from food to nourish our bodies and give us energy; toxic substances and waste products are excreted. The focus of this book and the site of LGS is the small intestine. In a healthy gut, the lining of the small intestine functions as a barrier made up of cells that are linked tightly together like bricks in a wall. When this lining is disrupted, small openings appear in the wall, which can allow the contents of the small intestine to escape from the GI tract into the blood stream.

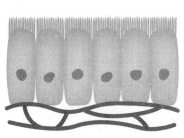 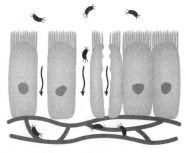

Normal, tight junction   Leaky and inflamed

FIGURE 1: Single cell intestinal lining

Leaky gut syndrome (LGS), also known as "intestinal permeability," happens when this lining is damaged. If this happens, partially digested proteins and toxins can be absorbed into the bloodstream. This causes inflammation and can trigger an immune response (the immune system attacks the proteins and toxins that it identifies as a danger). Sometimes, healthy cells and tissues get caught up in this response, resulting in autoimmune disease.

The bottom line is this: everything we eat impacts our nutritional and hormonal balance. Most patients I see with chronic illnesses are suffering from gut issues. The Standard American Diet (a.k.a. SAD), made up of too many refined and processed foods, soft drinks, and sugary desserts, is literally making us sick to our stomachs. This is why changing your diet is the best and fastest way to treat LGS and to alleviate the chronic conditions related to it.

Symptoms of Leaky Gut

One of the first signs that you may have a leaky gut is food sensitivities. The following are some other symptoms of LGS to look out for:

- Acid reflux
- Anxiety
- Bloating
- Diarrhea

- Headaches
- IBS
- Joint and muscle pain
- Low energy
- Skin issues, including rashes, rosacea, acne, eczema, and psoriasis
- Weight gain

If not repaired, intestinal permeability can potentially lead to more severe health issues, such as:

- Arthritis
- Autoimmune disorders
- Chronic fatigue
- Depression
- Migraines
- Multiple sclerosis (MS)
- Systemic lupus erythematosus (lupus, SLE)
- Type 1 diabetes

What Causes Leaky Gut?

Leaky gut can be caused by a number of factors, including:

- Alcohol use
- Frequent use of certain medications
- Genetic predisposition
- Poor diet
- Smoking

The most common dietary culprits that cause LGS include:

- **Casein.** Casein is a protein found in conventional cow's milk and dairy products such as cheese. My partners and I tested patients for dairy allergies and observed that over 80 percent of them had high antibody levels to casein. This means that when patients consumed casein-containing products, inflammation developed.

- **Gluten.** Gluten is a protein found in many grains such as wheat, rye, and barley. Gluten is difficult to digest and can damage your intestinal lining, depending on how well your body tolerates it. Approximately 20 percent of the patients we tested had high antibody levels to gluten.

- **Lectins.** Lectins (LEK tnz) are proteins found in many foods, not just grains; when they are consumed in small amounts, your body normally does just fine with them. But foods with large amounts of lectins are more problematic. Some of the foods containing lectins that cause leaky gut include wheat, rice, spelt, and soy.

- **Refined sugars.** Refined sugars depress the immune system and can sap the body of vitamins and minerals. Sugar can also feed the growth of yeast, including candida (a type of yeast that lives on and in the body), as well as bad bacteria, which further damages your gut. Bad bacteria actually create toxins called exotoxins that damage healthy cells and can eat a hole into your intestinal wall.

- **Soy.** Soy is highly allergenic—easily in the top 10 list of allergens. Ironically, soy is promoted as a safe alternative for those who have allergies to peanuts, dairy, and gluten. Even though you may not have a strong allergic reaction to soy, any allergen can contribute to leaky gut syndrome. More information about soy can be found in my book *The Soy Deception*.

I will explain more about the Gut Guzzlers listed above and why you should eliminate them from your diet in the next chapter, "The Heal Your Leaky Gut Diet." In the meantime, here are a few other important gut facts.

The Brain-Gut Connection

If you've ever "gone with your gut," felt "butterflies in your stomach" when anxious, or had a "gut-wrenching" experience, you are likely getting signals from your *second brain*. Research has shown that a lesser-known nervous system in the gut communicates with our brains. Together, these two brains play a key role when it comes to certain diseases in our bodies and to our overall health. This brain–gut connection is revolutionizing medicine's understanding of the links between digestion, mood, health, and even the way you think.

The scientific name for this other brain is the enteric nervous system (ENS). The ENS is composed of two thin layers of more than 100 million nerve cells lining your entire GI tract. As Jay Pasricha, MD, director of the Johns Hopkins Center for

Neurogastroenterology (the study of the brain and gut and their impact on GI disorders) explains, "The enteric nervous system doesn't seem capable of thought as we know it, but it communicates back and forth with our big brain—with profound results."

This communication between the brain and digestive system is opening up new ways of thinking about diseases. Not only do the gut and the brain communicate through the nervous system but also through hormones and the immune system. We know that microorganisms in the gut also help regulate the body's immune response. Medical researchers who study depression, Parkinson's disease, Alzheimer's disease, autism spectrum disorder (ASD), multiple sclerosis (MS), pain, anxiety, and other "neuro" conditions are now looking at what's going on in their patients' guts. Likewise, researchers who study ulcers, constipation, and other GI conditions focus on aspects of their patients' brain function. All this new information has given birth to a medical specialty called behavioral medicine, which holistic doctors heartily embrace.

Good Versus Bad Bacteria

The human gut has around 300 to 500 different strains of bacteria containing over 2 million genes! I know *bacteria* sounds like a bad word. But the bacterial population called the microbiome (mai kruh BAI owm) that lives in our intestine helps digest our food, regulate our immune system, and protect the cells in our gut from invading pathogens; the microbiome also promotes repair of damaged tissue. In other words, the good bacteria in your body prevent bad bacteria from growing and causing diseases.

As I mentioned, when helpful bacteria multiply and thrive in our bodies, they act as our protectors. At times, however, we put these beneficial bacteria at risk. One such instance is when we take antibiotics to treat an infection. Although an antibiotic kills the harmful bacteria causing the infection, it can also kill helpful bacteria that colonize our gut. This causes an imbalance of bacteria in the body that can lead to diarrhea and other gastrointestinal problems. Antibiotics are necessary to treat certain ailments, but they can wreak havoc on our gut and should not be overprescribed.

Other good bacteria include probiotic bacteria. Research has shown that the probiotic bacteria *Lactobacillus rhamnosus* contain the neurotransmitter GABA that can help regulate brain activity and calm anxiety. (Probiotics are live bacteria present in yogurts and other fermented foods.) A 2011 Irish university study of mice that consumed the probiotic found that the bacteria reduced stress by altering the rodents' brain chemistry. Research further shows that altering bacteria in the gut through specific diets may help treat neurodevelopmental disorders, including autism spectrum disorders and hyperactivity. Another recent study published in the journal *Nature Metabolism* found that as people get older, the composition of their gut microbiome tends to change. The greater the change, the better it is for your health and longevity.

The idea that certain types of bacteria can improve our health is not new, however. It has been around since the early 20th century, when Nobel Prize–winning biologist Élie Metchnikoff first proposed that eating bacteria similar to those living in the body could have health benefits. Probiotics (which means "for life") have these bacteria. Fortunately, probiotics and prebiotics (plant fibers that stimulate the growth of good bacteria in the gut) are available in many foods, beverages, and supplements. I use many of these in my practice, and I will tell you which are most gut-friendly later on.

Get Tested

I recommend that you take a leaky gut test before you start this diet to better identify the root cause of your symptoms and to help pinpoint potential contributing factors. The best test for this is a stool-sample analysis. I realize this sounds unpleasant, but it's an excellent way to diagnose malabsorption syndrome, which is poor nutrient absorption due to LGS. If you've never done this test before, ask your doctor for a stool-sample kit that you can take home. Follow the instructions carefully and mail the completed kit to the laboratory. The lab will do a microscopic examination and chemical tests that check for occult blood (blood that cannot be seen with the naked eye), fat, fibers, bile, white blood cells, and sugars. What's called a stool "culture" will identify whether you are properly digesting your food. The test can also check for the health of the intestines by identifying bacteria, both good and bad, as well as the presence of parasites and yeast. Once all this information is gathered, an individualized treatment and diet plan can be developed to help you and your gut get healthier. Remember to talk to your doctor about how to prepare for the test and what the results mean.

Turn the page when you're ready to take the first step of the Leaky Gut Diet and start your journey to good health!

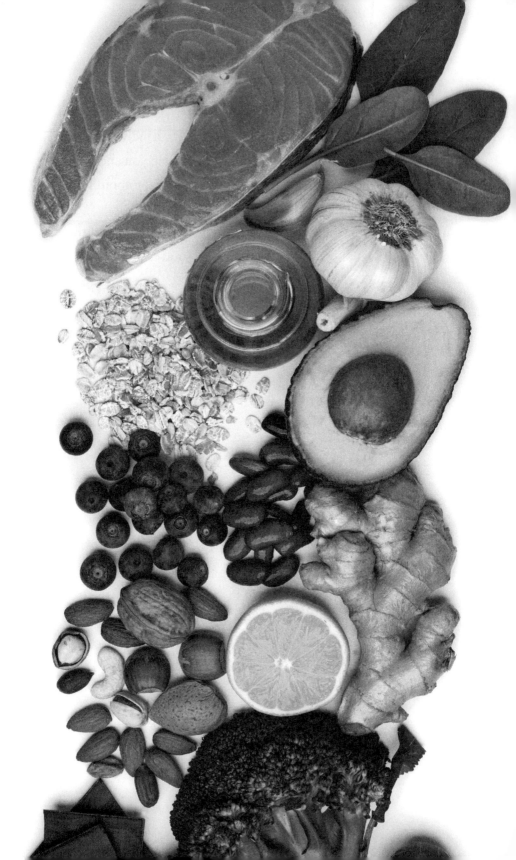

CHAPTER 2

The Heal Your Leaky Gut Diet

I like to tell my patients that changing their diet takes intestinal fortitude. That's right—it takes guts to clean up your gut! Eliminating some of your favorite foods and beverages can be tough, especially if they've brought you comfort. But there's a big payoff to following the Heal Your Leaky Gut Diet and Meal Plan. By following the steps outlined in this chapter, you will begin to feel better almost immediately, but it will likely take eight weeks (and sometimes longer) for your gut to fully heal. Think of it this way: It took however old you are now for your gut to get to the current condition it is in. What's another two months? In eight weeks, you will have gotten rid of the Gut Guzzlers that are making you sick and replaced them with healthier, tastier Good Gut foods and beverages. Here are the steps:

Step 1: Keep a Food and Symptom Diary

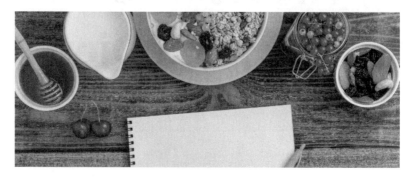

Being mindful of what you eat and drink each day and of the physical reactions/symptoms you have afterward will help you pinpoint what's causing your leaky gut. Keeping a food diary can help you understand which foods are helping and which may be causing problems. Studies have shown that recording food intake can help those who struggle with weight loss. In fact, researchers found that people who kept a food diary lost nearly twice as much weight as those who did not.

To be successful with a food diary, you have to record *everything* you eat and drink. The journal pages in the back of this book are there for you to track your progress. If you've already taken a leaky gut test and you know the types of foods your body is intolerant or allergic to, you can immediately remove those Gut Guzzlers from your diet. If not, record what you eat and drink before starting the diet and then throughout the next eight weeks. Remember to write down improvements (e.g., more energy, no stomach pain after breakfast, etc.) as well as symptoms. See the example food and symptom diary entry below:

HEAL YOUR LEAKY GUT DIET AND MEAL PLAN
DAILY FOOD AND SYMPTOMS DIARY

MEAL	TIME	FOOD/DRINK [+ amounts]	SYMPTOMS [bloating, abdominal pain, nausea, heartburn, diarrhea, brain fog, irritability, headache, etc.]	TIME & DURATION OF SYMPTOMS	OTHER FACTORS [stress, sleep, exercise, illness, medicines, remedies]
Breakfast	8 a.m.	frosted cornflakes, 1/2 cup whole milk, 1/2 cup orange juice, 8 oz	bloating, abdominal pain	2 hours	Woke up drowsy, restless night, took 2 Benadryl tablets at night
Morning Snack	10 a.m.	candy bar, 1.84 oz (52 g)	constipation	24 hours	
Lunch	Noon	cheeseburger, 4 oz (113 g) soda, 11 oz (325 mL)	headache, brain fog	3 hours	
Afternoon Snack	3 p.m.	small bag of potato chips, 1.5 oz (42.5 g)	bloating, stomachache		
Dinner	7 p.m.	frozen dinner, spaghetti with tomato sauce, 15 oz (425 g)	felt full after eating		Ate while watching TV
Evening Snack	10 p.m.	beer, 12 oz (355 mL)	cramping		Stressed about work
Notes					

Step 2: Goodbye Gut Guzzlers

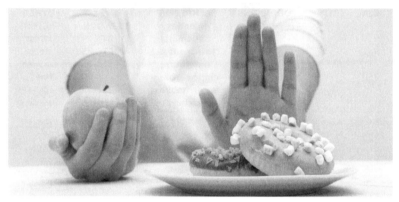

Healing your gut begins with removing the foods and ingredients that deplete vital nutrients from your body. Remember the Gut Guzzlers from the previous chapter? Some or all of the following are likely causing your LGS.

Ditch the Dairy

Dairy might be the granddaddy of all Gut Guzzlers. Here's why: As we age, many of us lose the ability to break down lactose, the main ingredient in milk. People with lactose intolerance do not have an allergy, but they are unable to digest lactose. An estimated 65 percent of the world's population is lactose intolerant. Lactose intolerance is not the only issue with dairy. As I mentioned earlier, the main milk protein associated with dairy allergies and LGS is casein. A casein allergy occurs when your body's immune system mistakenly thinks the casein protein is harmful and inappropriately produces antibodies for protection. Lactose-free milk still contains casein proteins, so if you have been diagnosed with a dairy allergy, lactose-free milk will still cause an allergic reaction.

Symptoms of both casein allergy and lactose intolerance include bloating; pain; gas; diarrhea; gastroesophageal reflux (stomach contents rise up into the esophagus); swollen lips, tongue, and throat; skin rash; coughing; wheezing; nasal congestion; and runny nose. Feeling sluggish? Dairy might have something to do with that too. If you need more reasons to cut out dairy, consider the fact that it is not a necessary part of a healthy adult diet. Giving up milk doesn't mean doing without calcium. Plenty of foods are good sources of calcium, including leafy greens, vegetables, nuts, seeds, beans, lean locally-farmed meats, pasture-raised poultry, and wild-raised seafood. To go casein-free, you need to eliminate cow's milk found in:

- Baked goods that contain milk
- Buttermilk
- Cheese
- Chocolate (white, milk, or dark)
- Cottage cheese
- Cream
- Creamed soups
- Ice cream
- Milk
- Sour cream
- Yogurt made with cow's milk

While these are the major sources of dairy, lactose and casein can be hiding in other foods, including:

- Butter
- Curds
- Dry milk powder
- Margarines
- Milk byproducts
- Non-fat dry milk
- Recaldent (in gum, mints, and toothpaste)
- Shortening

GO WITH YOUR GUT TIP

Read the Label

Manufacturers in the United States must list on the label whether a food contains any of the most common allergens. If a food contains casein, for example, the label should clearly say "contains milk ingredients," "made with milk ingredients," or "processed in a facility that also processes milk products." Always read the label before buying.

Alternative Names for Casein

When reading labels, look out for these ingredients that contain casein:

- Caseinate
- Casein hydrolysate
- Fortified proteins
- Milk protein

- Milk solids
- Paracasein
- Rennet casein

Goodbye Gluten

Another common condition I find in my patients with LGS is gluten allergy. Gluten is a protein naturally found in grains such as wheat, barley, and rye. Gluten acts as a binder that holds food together; it's what makes pizza dough stretchy. Without gluten, the dough would fall apart. Gluten is also sold as wheat gluten, or seitan (SAY tan), a popular vegan high-protein food. Lesser-known sources of gluten include soy sauce and modified food starch.

The problem with gluten is that it can cause serious side effects. For some people, the body interprets gluten as a toxin, causing the immune cells to overreact and attack it. This results in inflammation. Symptoms can range from mild fatigue, rashes, bloating, and alternating constipation and diarrhea, to unintended weight loss, malnutrition, and intestinal damage. The most severe cases are related to celiac disease, which is an autoimmune disorder.

It is estimated that 1 in 133 Americans have celiac disease, and around 83 percent of them are undiagnosed or misdiagnosed with other conditions. Research shows that people with celiac disease have a higher risk of osteoporosis and anemia due to malabsorption of calcium and iron, respectively; infertility;

nerve disorders; and, in rare cases, cancer. The good news is that removing gluten from the diet can allow the intestines to reverse the damage. If you are allergic to gluten or have celiac disease, you should plan to eliminate the following foods from your diet.

Grains

These grains contain gluten:

- Barley
- Bulger
- Couscous
- Durum
- Einkorn
- Emmer
- Farina
- Farro
- Graham
- Kamut
- Khorasan
- Malt
- Rye
- Semolina
- Spelt
- Triticale (a blend of wheat and rye)
- Wheat bran
- Wheat berries
- Wheat germ
- Wheat starch

Breads

Most breads, crackers, and wraps contain gluten. The only way to know for sure is to *read the ingredients list* and check to see which grains are used. If you have a gluten intolerance, avoid the following:

- Bagels
- Flatbread
- Flour tortillas
- Potato bread
- Rye
- Sourdough

- Wheat crackers
- White bread
- Whole wheat bread
- Whole wheat wraps

Condiments

Many popular condiments also contain gluten. These include:

- Soy sauce
- Barbecue sauce
- Salad dressings
- Marinades
- Cream sauces
- Spice blends
- Gravy mixes
- Malt vinegar
- Ketchup

Baked Goods

Baked goods are typically made with wheat flour or other gluten-containing grains. Because of this, people with a gluten intolerance should largely avoid the following:

- Cakes
- Cookies
- Doughnuts
- Pancakes
- Pastries
- Pretzels (soft and hard)
- Muffins
- Waffles

Wheat-Based Pastas

Pastas are a staple in many cultures and one of the most beloved comfort foods. Although most traditional pastas are made with gluten-containing grains, gluten-free alternatives are readily available. Pastas to avoid include:

- Dumplings
- Gnocchi made with wheat flour

- Spaghetti

Processed Foods

Processed foods in general are on the no-fly list for people trying to heal a leaky gut. Those with celiac disease should be especially careful to avoid the following:

- Canned soups and soup mixes
- Cereals
- Egg substitutes
- French fries and other fried foods
- Meat substitutes, such as veggie burgers and hot dogs
- Prepared lunch meats
- Processed cheeses
- Puddings and instant dessert mixes

> **GO WITH YOUR GUT TIP**
>
> ### Gluten-Free Doesn't Mean Nutrient-Dense
>
> The gluten-free food market has grown into a multi-billion-dollar industry with a host of products now sold in most supermarkets. This includes gluten-free cookies, chips, and other snack foods. But beware of the generally low nutritional quality of processed gluten-free foods! Highly processed gluten-free alternatives may contain refined sugars and saturated fats and have a higher glycemic (glayh SEE mihk) index than their gluten-full counterparts. The glycemic index measures how quickly carbohydrates enter the bloodstream as glucose. (See chart, for example, here: https://universityhealthnews.com/

daily/nutrition/glycemic-index-chart/) More often than not, these gluten-free foods are made with processed unfortified rice, tapioca, corn, or potato flours. Whole grains with gluten have fiber and nutrients, including B vitamins, magnesium, and iron, which gluten-free alternatives frequently lack. To make up for these important missing nutrients, eat naturally gluten-free foods in their whole form such as fruits, vegetables, nuts, seeds, fish, eggs, and poultry.

Shun the Sugar

Getting my patients to lay off sweets is probably the most difficult task I have as a doctor.

Today, the average American consumes nearly 152 pounds of sugar annually.

Refined sugar is the worst offender because it's made from sugarcane or sugar beets that are stripped of vitamins, minerals, and nutrients. To properly digest excess sugar, the body must use its own store of nutrients, particularly B vitamins. Sugar also wreaks havoc in your gut by feeding bad gut bacteria that cause LGS. Talk about a Gut Guzzler!

While we sometimes knowingly add sugar to food, we are largely unaware that most of the sugar we consume comes from processed and prepared foods. Sugar-sweetened beverages and breakfast cereals are two of the worst offenders. Research clearly shows that refined sugar seriously damages health, leading to weight gain, high blood pressure, and spiked cholesterol levels—just for starters. Sugar also depresses the immune system and elevates the body's own blood-sugar levels, putting people at risk for diabetes; heart, liver, and kidney disease; arthritis; and osteoporosis. One study published in the journal *Circulation* showed that sugar-sweetened drinks directly cause cardiovascular disease and diabetes that kills about 184,000 people worldwide every year.

Examples of refined sugars:

- Brown sugar
- High fructose corn syrup
- Powdered sugar
- Turbinado sugar
- White sugar

Are You a Sugar Addict?

Do you find that you can't make it through the day without at least one can of Coke? Do you crave a sweet treat after every meal? Sugar addiction is real. Once you're hooked, cravings can be hard to resist, leading you down a slippery slope toward chronic health problems. Studies show that in some people and animals, the brain reacts to sugar much like it does to drugs and alcohol, which is why it's so difficult to quit. Rest assured, your efforts to cut out refined sugar will pay off in the long run. If you stick to your sugar detox, you will notice you have more energy and less fatigue. Your cravings will eventually stop, your risk of illness and disease will diminish, and your leaky gut will heal.

GO WITH YOUR GUT TIP
The Sweet Smell of Success

Believe it or not, eating isn't the only way to feel sated, or full. When our nose detects sweet smells, the appetite-control center in our brain receives a message that food has been consumed—even if we haven't taken a bite. So, the next time you crave a sweet treat, try inhaling pure vanilla extract or vanilla essential oil to cut your cravings. You can smell it directly from the bottle or place a few drops on a cloth and sniff it throughout the day. Ideally, smell the scent at least three times a day for 30 seconds each time.

Symptoms of Hyperglycemia (High Blood Sugar)

Hyperglycemia, the precursor to diabetes and other conditions, occurs when you have too much glucose (sugar) in your blood. Symptoms to watch out for:

- Fruity smelling breath
- Fatigue and weakness
- Headache or brain fog
- Blurred vision
- Increased thirst and urination

Glycemic Index

The glycemic index measures how quickly carbohydrates enter the bloodstream as glucose. (See chart, for example, here: https://universityhealthnews.com/daily/nutrition/glycemic-index-chart/)

GO WITH YOUR GUT TIP

Sugar Detox

There's more than one way to do a sugar detox. Some of my patients feel the need to go cold turkey. But for most people, I recommend weaning off sugar gradually, one meal or snack at a time. You will find that your palate will adjust to less sweetness over time and that your cravings will soon disappear.

Lectins

Lectins are proteins that bind to carbohydrates. They are found mainly in legumes and grains. Some lectins are harmless, and others, such as those in kidney beans, can cause digestive symptoms if not cooked properly. Lectins can also negatively affect people who have digestive sensitivities or gastrointestinal distress. The reason for this is that lectins may interfere with both the gut microbiota and the absorption of nutrients. In addition, lectins may decrease acid secretion and increase inflammation. Lectins are present in most plant foods but are especially high in the following:

- Grains, such as barley, quinoa, and rice
- Legumes, such as beans, lentils, peas, soybeans, and peanuts
- Nightshade vegetables (a family of plants that includes tomatoes, eggplant, potatoes, and peppers)

For many foods containing harmful lectins, such as kidney beans, cooking greatly reduces their lectin content, making them safe to eat. It's a good idea to boil beans for 30 minutes to eliminate their harmful lectins. Soaking beans also reduces their lectin content, though perhaps not enough to ensure safety. Foods that contain lectins are often full of antioxidants, vitamins, and minerals that are good for you. If you are not lectin-sensitive, these benefits will likely outweigh the negative effects of lectins to the body. If you are allergic or have food sensitivities, however, I recommend reducing the lectins in your diet or eliminating them entirely.

Stop the Soy

Soy is often touted as the ultimate health food and is used as a substitute for milk and meat. Nothing could be further from the truth. Studies showing soy's adverse effects on the thyroid date back 75 years. Soy consumption inhibits the uptake of iodine, which is used by the thyroid gland in the production of thyroid hormones. It can cause goiter, which is swelling of the thyroid gland. Another problem with soy is that it contains phytoestrogens, chemicals that mimic estrogen hormones. I also have good reason to believe soy can contribute to hormone-sensitive cancers such as breast, uterine, ovarian, prostate, and testicular cancers.

The phosphates in soy hinder the body's ability to assimilate important minerals such as calcium, copper, iron, magnesium, and zinc. Soy also interferes with the production of vitamin D and can cause a vitamin B12 deficiency. Additionally, soy is an extremely allergic food source. In my practice, I have found that many patients who have a milk allergy are also allergic to soy.

Step 3: Good Gut Substitutes

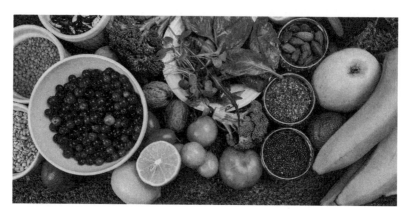

The third step on the Heal Your Leaky Gut Diet is to replace the Gut Guzzlers with Good Gut foods. Use this chart to find healthier replacements.

Instead of Cow's Milk:

For those who are lactose intolerant, lactose-free milk is treated with the enzyme lactase to break down the lactose. It is closest to regular cow's milk in taste and offers the same nutrients, such as calcium. Other Good Gut non-cow's milk options include these:

- Almond
- Cashew
- Coconut
- Hazelnut
- Hemp
- Oat
- Rice

Note: I do not recommend soy milk as a substitute for the reasons I stated earlier. And the above products should be unsweetened.

Instead of regular ice cream:
- Almond-based frozen desserts
- Coconut ice cream
- Rice ice cream

Instead of cow's milk yogurt:
- Coconut yogurt
- Oat yogurt
- Rice yogurt

Instead of cow's milk powder:
- Coconut powder

Instead of gluten-containing grains:
- Amaranth
- Arrowroot
- Brown, black, or red rice
- Buckwheat
- Corn
- Gluten-free oats
- Millet
- Quinoa
- Sorghum

- Teff

Instead of wheat flour and gluten-containing breads:
- Corn tortillas
- Gluten-free multiseed
- Rye (rye bread is rich in fiber)
- Sourdough
- Sprouted grain

Instead of refined sugar:
Natural sugars are less harmful than artificial sugars and even have health benefits. Examples of natural sugars include:
- Agave nectar (extracted from core of the agave plant)
- Coconut palm sugar
- Raw honey
- Maple sugar (dehydrated maple syrup)
- Maple syrup (good source of manganese, zinc, and other nutrients)
- Molasses (blackstrap molasses is a great source of iron, calcium, copper, potassium, and magnesium)
- Rapadura (unrefined and unbleached whole cane sugar)
- Sucanat® (does not have the molasses removed, so it retains nutrient value)

Stevia is a healthy artificial sugar option, followed by xylitol, erythritol, and yacon syrup:

- Stevia (an herb that comes in powder extract or liquid concentrate)
- Xylitol (a low-glycemic sweetener that's safe for people with diabetes or hypoglycemia)
- Erythritol (an organic sugar alcohol used as a sugar substitute)
- Yacon syrup (a natural sweetening agent extracted from the roots of the yacon plant)

Conversion for 1 cup of white sugar

These substitutions will help when making recipes that call for refined sugar.

Coconut palm sugar	1 to 1 replacement, white or brown sugar
Honey (raw)	⅔ cup; reduce liquids in recipe by ¼ cup
Maple sugar	¾ cup
Maple syrup	¾ cup; reduce liquids in recipe by 3 tbsp
Molasses (blackstrap)	⅔ cup; reduce liquids in recipe by 5 tbsp
Rapadura	1 to 1 replacement, white or brown sugar
Stevia	⅛ –¼ tsp
Sucanat	1 to 1 replacement; white or brown sugar
Xylitol	1 to 1 replacement, white or brown sugar

Rule of thumb: If substituting a liquid form of sweetener for a dry form, either decrease the liquids in the recipe by ¼ cup for every cup of sweetener that you use or add ¼ cup of flour.

Instead of sweetened cereals:

Steel-cut oats, homemade pancakes/waffles with whole grains

Instead of cakes, cookies, candies, and sweet desserts:

Fresh fruit

Instead of canned fruits that contain syrups, salts, and preservatives:

- Fresh or frozen fruits

Instead of sodas:

- Coconut water
- Fruit-infused sparkling water
- Freshly squeezed lemonade with honey or agave nectar
- Kombucha

Instead of regular cheese:

- Nut cheese
- Rice cheese

Note: Cheeses must be casein-free and whey-free.

Instead of white rice, use organic sources of:

- Brown rice
- Broccoli rice
- Riced cauliflower
- Riced broccoli
- Shirataki rice
- Wild rice

GO WITH YOUR GUT TIP

Creamy Without Cream

To thicken soups and sauces without cream, add soaked and puréed cashews. For creamier salad dressing, use coconut milk.

Instead of regular chocolate:

Dairy-free chocolate and chocolate chips

Instead of butter:

Coconut oil or ghee (approximately ⅞ cup to 1 cup butter)

Instead of refined table salt:

- Crodarom™ Bali Sea Salt
- Celtic Sea Salt
- Eden Sea Salt
- Halen Môn Pure Sea Salt (from Britain)
- Hawaiian red Alaea salt
- Himalayan Crystal Salt
- Mineral Mountain Krystal Salt® (from the Himalayas)

- Redmond Real Salt (from Utah)

When Baking:

Instead of butter or oil:
Mashed banana, applesauce, nut butters, or cooked pumpkin

Instead of bouillon cubes:
Stocks from grass-fed and/or organic beef, chicken, turkey, and fish

Instead of commercial sausage, lunch meats, smoked meats, and animals bred in factory farms in confinement and given antibiotics or hormones:
Grass-fed, organic, and antibiotic/hormone-free meat and poultry

Instead of regular supermarket eggs:
Organic, pasture-raised/free-range, certified humane eggs (Shell color makes no difference. Note that "cage-free" does not mean free-range. Fertile eggs have the most nutrients.)

Instead of imported cod, grouper, orange roughy, sea bass, red snapper, swordfish, shark, tilefish, catfish, farmed salmon, fish canned in vegetable oils, fried fish, or frozen

fish sticks:

Fresh and wild caught from the ocean: Arctic char, wild Alaskan salmon, sardines, anchovies, Dungeness and stone crab, Pacific halibut, clams, mussels, oysters, herring, lobster (from California or Florida), tuna, pink shrimp, US farmed tilapia, rainbow trout, farmed scallops

Step 4: Hydrate

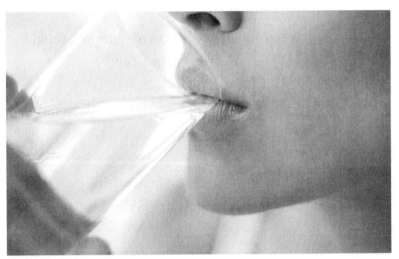

The fourth step to healing your gut is maintaining optimal hydration. A key element of the Heal Your Leaky Gut Diet is drinking more water. However much water you drink now, I can almost guarantee you it is not enough. The one symptom I see in just about all of my patients is dehydration, a leading cause of digestive and other health problems. Soda and juice don't hydrate you like water does. They can even enhance dehydration, and I'll explain why later on. Your beverage of choice should always be water. If the water in your area is not great, I suggest getting a water filter. (PUR® or Brita® are the best.)

Rather than estimating the number of glasses you should drink a day, use the easy calculation below. It will tell you exactly how much water is needed for adequate hydration at your weight:

Weight/Water Calculation

- Take your weight in pounds.
- Divide that number by 2.
- The result is the number of ounces of water you should drink daily. (There are 8 ounces in 1 cup.)

Let's say Janice weighs 130 pounds. The math would look like this:

- 130/2 = 65 ounces
- How many cups of water should Janice drink each day?
- 65/8 = 8.125, so a little over 8 cups per day

Keep in mind that the human body is 60 percent water, while the brain is about 70 percent water.

Drop the Pop

I've explained how refined sugar can adversely affect your health. One of the biggest sources of sugar for many people is what they drink: sodas, fruit juices, highly sweetened coffees, and other sweet beverages. Soft drinks are a leading cause of obesity because drinking carbonated sugary drinks does not make you feel full. Not surprisingly, studies show that people who drink sugar-sweetened beverages consistently gain more weight than people who don't. In one study of children, each daily serving of sugar-sweetened beverages was linked to a 60 percent increased risk of obesity.

The Bad Juju in Juice

Many people believe that fruit juice is healthier than soda, but the truth is they both pack around 20 to 26 grams of sugar per cup. Because of its high sugar content, juice should be avoided just as much as a Big Gulp. Apple juice is particularly high in sugar, and a 2012 study published in the *Journal of Environmental Health* found 32 percent of the apple juices tested had unacceptable levels of arsenic that can damage the brain and heart.

Additionally, some people have difficulty digesting fructose, the main sugar in fruit. Fructose intolerance affects about 1 in 130,000 people, according to the *Journal of Nutrition and Metabolism*. Symptoms include stomach pain, bloating, and diarrhea, making juice a Gut Guzzler for some. That said, if you are not fructose intolerant, it's always better to eat an apple or an orange than to drink it in juice form.

Step 5: Eat Mindfully

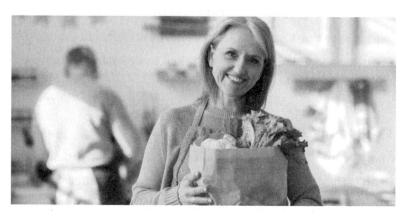

This step requires you to be mindful of what and how you are eating. Are you the first person to clean your plate at the dinner table? Have you been known to "inhale" your food? If so, chances are you are eating too fast and not chewing your food thoroughly, which could be contributing to your intestinal distress. The combination of taking smaller bites and chewing properly breaks down food better and activates enzymes in your mouth that aid digestion.

Being mindful of how and what you are eating helps you fully savor your meals and feel full. When we eat on the run or while reading, watching TV, or texting, we tend to consume too much too quickly. Remember the brain-gut connection? When we eat, it takes 20 minutes for our brain to realize that we are full. Being distracted when eating prevents us from getting that message. In essence, mindful eating means being fully attentive to your food, including when you buy, prepare, serve, and consume it.

Adopting this new attitude toward food and meals might take some practice, but it's worth it. Here are some suggestions:

1. Begin with your shopping list (see page 47). Consider the health value of every item you add to your list and stick to your list to avoid impulse buying. Fill most of your shopping cart in the produce section and avoid the center aisles, which are heavily stocked with processed foods. Watch out for the chips and candy at the checkout counter.

2. Come to the table with an appetite—but not when ravenously hungry. When we skip meals, we tend to eat too quickly at the next one. Satisfying hunger becomes the priority, rather than enjoying our food.

3. Start with a smaller portion. When you eat mindfully, you may not need or want a full plate of food. It's possible that your "eyes are bigger than your stomach." You can always go back for seconds if you're still hungry. (See page 140 for portion-size tips.)

4. Appreciate your food. Pause for a moment before you begin eating to contemplate the meal on your table. Silently express your gratitude for the opportunity to enjoy delicious food with your family members or eating companions. Saying a blessing before meals is a formal expression of gratitude and a tradition in many religions, including Christianity, Judaism, Islam, and Hinduism.

5. Bring all your senses to the meal. When you're cooking, serving, and eating your food, be aware of its color, texture, and aroma. If you are eating out at a fine restaurant,

observe the plating of your food (how it's presented on your plate). Think about the bubbling, sizzling sounds you hear while preparing the food. Another way to eat mindfully is to try identifying the ingredients and seasonings that went into your meal by flavor: citrus, acidic, savory, sweet, spicy.

6. Take small bites. It's easier to taste food completely when your mouth isn't full. A good way to stop yourself from eating too quickly is to put down your fork or spoon between bites. You can also take half a forkful or half a spoonful.

7. Chew thoroughly. A rule of thumb is to chew each bite 32 times (on average, depending on what you are eating) so that you can taste the essence of the food. You may be surprised at all the flavors that are released.

8. Don't talk with your mouth full. Your mother was right! In addition to being considered rude, talking while eating doesn't allow you to chew your food properly. When eating with companions, allow time for conversation, when one person is eating and listening while the other is speaking. If you follow the advice above, you won't scarf your food down.

Step 6: Move

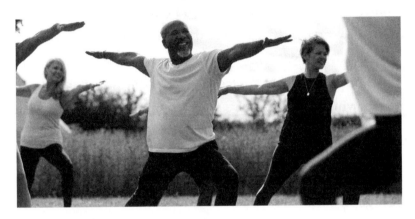

The final step in the Heal Your Leaky Gut Diet isn't about food or diet, but you can do this step from day one. Studies after studies clearly show that physical activity boosts immune function, decreases inflammation, and encourages the growth of new blood vessels in both the brain and the body. Exercise promotes weight loss and increases good cholesterol (HDL) while lowering blood pressure, bad cholesterol (LDL), and blood sugar (glucose) levels.

I realize that many people hate to exercise. But movement is the goal, not running a marathon or working out six days a week at a gym (although neither of those is a bad thing as long as you are healthy and uninjured). If you have a sedentary lifestyle, the trick is finding an activity that you can start and stick with. The following strategies are for people of all fitness levels. As always, check with your doctor before starting any new exercise program.

Release Your Inner Athlete

Is there a sport or activity that you once enjoyed but haven't done in years? Maybe you used to swim, hike, bike, or play basketball. Did you play volleyball or soccer when you were in school? Remember the feeling of breathless excitement you had playing sports? Explore the possibilities. Join a local team or meetup. We tend to stick with activities that are fun rather than those we consider an obligation. Plus, we know exercise improves our mood thanks to endorphins, our body's natural feel-good hormones.

Walk It Off

Something as simple as a daily brisk walk can do wonders for your physical and mental health. The faster, farther, and more frequently you walk, the greater the benefits, but any movement is good for you. If you've been sedentary up until now, you may want to start at a slower pace and work your way up to walking faster and for longer distances. Pumping your arms back and forth as you walk will also bring up your heart rate. Power walking is a great way to get cardio activity, improve your heart health, and increase your endurance. You can also alternate periods of brisk walking with leisurely walking. This type of interval training helps improve cardiovascular fitness and burns more calories than regular walking.

Lift Weights, Lift Your Spirit

Did you know that weight lifting burns calories? Lifting weights (also called body sculpting or resistance training) can actually help you to slim down. Whether it's lifting hand weights at home or doing the machine circuit or barbells at the gym, resistance training can also improve your mood and bone health and increase your metabolism. In a 2017 study published in the journal *Sports Medicine*, researchers conducted a meta-analysis of 16 studies involving 992 participants; the study concluded that resistance training "significantly improves anxiety symptoms among both healthy participants and participants with a physical or mental illness."

GO WITH YOUR GUT TIP

How to Get Moving

Need some motivation to get moving? Enlist a walking buddy for your constitutionals or join/start a walking group. If you are the competitive type, challenge your friends to a walk-off. Use your smartphone or fitness watch to count the steps you take in one day. The winner with the most steps can buy the other person a 10-minute chair massage.

Plan Your Routine

Before you start your walking regimen, remember to:

- **Gear up.** Choose shoes with proper arch support, a firm heel, and thick flexible soles to cushion your feet and absorb shock. Wear comfortable, loose-fitting clothes and gear that's appropriate for all types of weather, such as layers in cooler weather. Wear moisture-wicking fabrics, which will keep you more comfortable. If you walk outdoors when it's dark, wear bright colors or reflective tape for visibility. Wear sunscreen, a hat, and sunglasses if you're going out during the day.

- **Choose your course carefully.** If you're walking outdoors, avoid paths with cracked sidewalks, potholes, low-hanging limbs, or uneven turf. After dark, choose well-lit routes. In inclement weather, consider walking in a shopping mall or other indoor public spaces.
- **Stay mindful.** Pay attention to your surroundings. If you wear ear buds or headphones, keep the volume down or leave one ear exposed to listen for traffic, other pedestrians, and animals.
- **Warm up.** Walk slowly for 5 to 10 minutes to warm up your muscles.
- **Cool down.** When you've been power walking and have broken a sweat, walk more slowly for 5 to 10 minutes when you're done to help your muscles cool down.
- **Stretch.** After you cool down, gently stretch your muscles.

Dance

Whether it's ballroom, tap, two-step, modern, hip-hop, or Zumba®, dancing is a fun way to get moving. Sign up for lessons or use one of the many online videos to dance as if no one's watching.

Walk the Dog

If the idea of power walking doesn't appeal to you, taking your four-legged friend on a few laps around the block or neighborhood will give you a chance to take in the fresh air and bond with your pooch.

Do Some Chores

For those who find exercise a chore, do some real work around the house or apartment instead. Washing your car and vacuuming the floors will actually get the heart rate pumping.

Garden and Yard Work

If you live in a house, gardening, raking leaves, and mowing the lawn (on foot) are good for the body and soul. Start a vegetable garden and use the harvest when making meals.

Work Out While Watching TV

Listen up, couch potatoes! Keep some hand weights near your sofa or chair and do a few arm curls while you're streaming your favorite series or movie. You can do leg lifts when sitting.

Get Up from Your Desk

If your work involves sitting at a desk or computer for eight hours a day, take breaks from your chair throughout the day by simply standing up or walking into another room. Set a timer as a reminder (every 20 or 30 minutes).

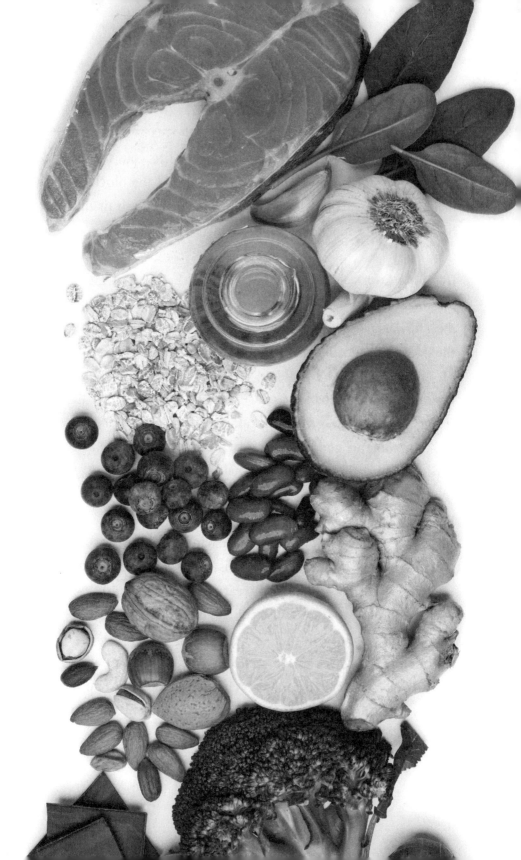

CHAPTER 3

Your Diet and Meal Plan

Planning your meals ahead of time is one of the most important things you can do to follow the Heal Your Leaky Gut Diet. Knowing what you're going to eat for the week saves time and energy in the long run and helps you resist the temptation to grab some fast food on the way home from work or after picking the kids up from school. You can cut down on the time it takes to grocery shop and have better control of your spending by buying exactly what you need for the upcoming week. Choose from the recipes in this book or experiment with your own healthy creations. Below is a sample meal planner you can use. Don't forget to write down what you need to take out of the freezer to thaw so that you don't end up with frozen food for dinner.

Weekly Meal Planner

	Breakfast	Lunch	Dinner	Snack
Monday				
Tuesday				
Wednesday				
Thursday				
Friday				
Saturday				
Sunday				

Shopping List

Meal Planning Tips

Plan weekly meals on Sundays

Pick a day to plan your meals for each week. On Sunday, for example, write down what you want to eat for breakfasts, lunches, and dinners. Figure out what ingredients you will need and make a shopping list. [See page 47 for a shopping list.] You might even cook on Sunday, freeze meal-sized portions, and enjoy leftovers during the week.

Prepare meals in the evening

Another idea is to set aside 15 to 20 minutes each weekday evening to prepare the meals for the following day. If you're too tired to cook full meals, do the prep work—mixing, soaking, chopping, or thawing—to get a head start. The more you do the night before, the less you will have to do after you get home from work!

BYO lunch and snacks

Buy a small soft-pack cooler to pack the leftovers, soups, salads, or whatever you've already prepared to bring with you for lunch. Put some nuts, dairy- and sugar-free yogurt, fruits, or vegetables in small, reusable containers for easy, healthy snacking.

Wake up 15 minutes earlier to make breakfast

Eating breakfast kick-starts your metabolism and gives you the energy to get things done and to focus at work or at school. Set aside 15 minutes each morning to make breakfast. Remember to include some healthy fat for energy throughout the morning. Avoid sugar and high-carb breakfasts that, aside from being Gut Guzzlers, will cause your blood sugar to crash before lunchtime. Look at the breakfast recipes in this book for ideas. A simple smoothie made with yogurt and kefir (dairy- and sugar-free) or coconut milk as a base is a quick and delicious way to start your day!

Use your phone calendar to schedule meals

Food should never be an afterthought. Use your smartphone calendar to notify you when it's time to plan, prepare, shop, and eat. Scheduling meals will keep you from skipping them, which makes you hungry and more likely to overeat or eat the wrong things.

Make more of your favorite meals

Whether you're cooking for one or for five, doubling or tripling a recipe will give you plenty of leftovers for meals the next day or, if you freeze, the following week.

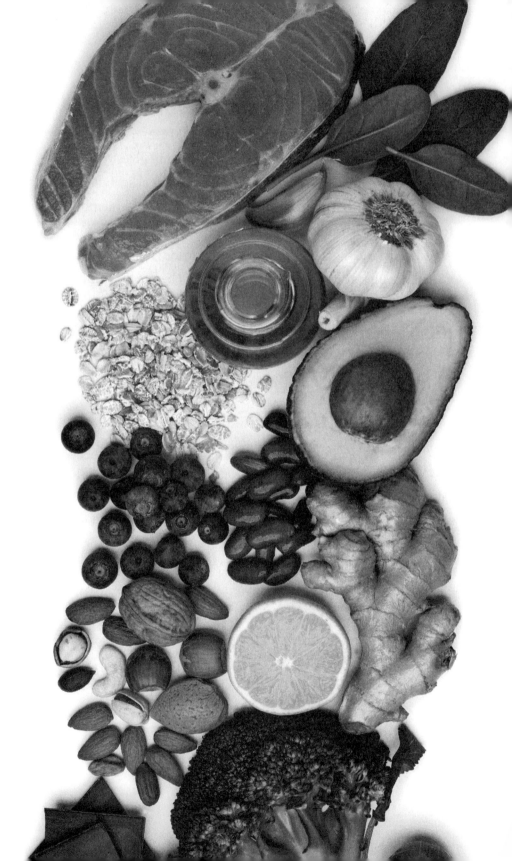

CHAPTER 4

The Heal Your Leaky Gut Weekly Meal Plan and Guide

Below is a sample seven-day menu plan to help you get started, along with a recap of general food and lifestyle tips to help kickstart your gut-healthy diet. (These are just suggestions, of course. You can pick and choose your favorite recipes in this book.) I've included some additional gut-friendly snacks that you can find in your new, well-stocked pantry.

Monday
Breakfast: Blueberry Muffins (p. 72)
Lunch: Crispy Chicken Salad with Lemon Raspberry Vinaigrette (p. 74)
Dinner: Sausage and Vegetable Bake (p. 80)
Snack: Zucchini Sticks (p. 76)

Dessert (optional): Coconut Cacao Bites (p. 105)

Tuesday
Breakfast: Crustless Veggie Quiche Cups (p. 73)
Lunch: Lemon Tahini Kale Salad (p. 93)
Dinner: Super Sloppy Joes (p. 96)
Snack: Pistachio and Hemp Seed Trail Mix (p. 101)
Dessert (optional): Berry sorbet

Wednesday
Breakfast: Coconut Mango Smoothie (p. 103) or Blueberry Muffins
Lunch: Taco Salad (p. 97)
Dinner: Chicken Fingers (p. 95) with veggie of your choice
Snack: Date Oat Bar
Dessert (optional): Peach Coconut Milk Ice Cream (p. 106)

Thursday
Breakfast: Spinach Omelet with homemade toast (Easy Delicious Bread, p. 102)
Lunch: Yogurt Ranch Vegetable Dip (p. 99)
Dinner: Salmon with Pecan Crust (p. 88), with veggie of your choice
Snack: Fruit Salad (5 strawberries, ¼ cup melon, ⅓ cup grapes)
Dessert (optional): Trader Joe's Soft-Baked Snickerdoodles® (dusted with cinnamon; wheat-, milk-, peanut-, tree nut-, and soy-free)

Friday

Breakfast: Homemade pancakes/waffles with whole grains (with pure maple syrup)

Lunch: Creamy Coconut Balsamic Salad with Brussels Sprouts, Walnuts, and Cranberries (p. 90)

Dinner: Honey Mustard Pork with Jicama and Green Apples (p. 84), and veggie of your choice

Snack: Dairy-free coconut yogurt (with blueberries)

Dessert (optional): Nutty Fruit Cobbler with Cashew Cream (p. 107)

Saturday

Breakfast: Steel-cut oatmeal with fresh fruit topping

Lunch: Creamy Chicken and Basil (p. 89)

Dinner: Vegetable Rice Stir-Fry (p. 83)

Snack: Sweet Potato Fries (p. 92)

Dessert (optional): Coconut milk pudding

Sunday

Breakfast: French toast with gluten-free sourdough bread, milk substitute, sliced bananas, sliced almonds, pure maple syrup

Lunch: Roasted chicken (seasoned with black pepper, fresh oregano, and fresh parsley)

Dinner: Beef and Vegetable Stew (p. 82) with cauliflower rice

Snack: Avocado and Almond Fruit Smoothie (p. 103)

Dessert (optional): Sugar-free, dairy-free frozen banana "ice cream" (Put four frozen bananas in a blender with a few teaspoons of dairy-free milk. Blend and enjoy!)

Your Gut-Healthy Diet Guide

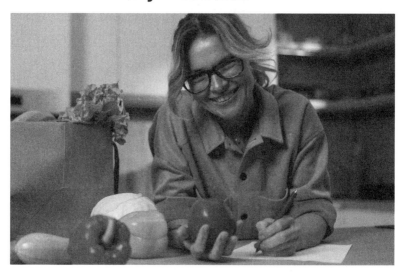

Here is a recap of the six steps on your journey to health and healing. (Refer to Chapter 2 for details on each step.)

- Step 1: Keep a Food and Symptom Diary (see p. 13 for templates)
- Step 2: Get Rid of Gut Guzzlers (Dairy, Gluten, Sugar, Lectins)
- Step 3: Substitute Good Gut Foods
- Step 4: Hydrate (with tap or bottled water, not soda/ sparkling water, seltzer, or juice)
- Step 5: Eat Mindfully

- Step 6: Move

Best Practices for a Better Gut:
- Avoid processed foods.
- Avoid foods high in hydrogenated "trans" fats (naturally occurring unsaturated fats found in milk and meat) and refined sugar.
- Eat whole and fermented foods, including vegetables, fruit, fish, eggs, nuts, seeds, and non-dairy yogurt, that support the growth of beneficial gut microbes.
- Drink adequate amounts of water and don't let yourself become dehydrated.
- Adopt healthy lifestyle habits, including exercise, meditation, and relaxation techniques (e.g., deep breathing, creative outlets).
- Get enough restorative sleep. (Avoid sleep medications.)
- Stop smoking and avoid secondhand smoke.
- Limit or avoid alcohol consumption.
- If you have a craving for sweets, satisfy it by choosing dark chocolate (at least 90 percent) in moderation. Dark chocolate isn't as sweet as milk chocolate, and it's packed with antioxidants and anti-inflammatory chemicals.
- Eat foods that are high in antioxidants, such as broccoli, spinach, carrots, and pumpkin. These foods help reduce the damage that is caused by the inflammatory process, including damage on a cellular level.

- Use natural anti-inflammatory herbs and spices such as turmeric, ginger, cinnamon, and chili powder.
- Fight inflammation naturally by consuming healthy fats and fat-rich fish, such as salmon, sardines, cod, and lake trout, which are high in omega-3 fatty acids.

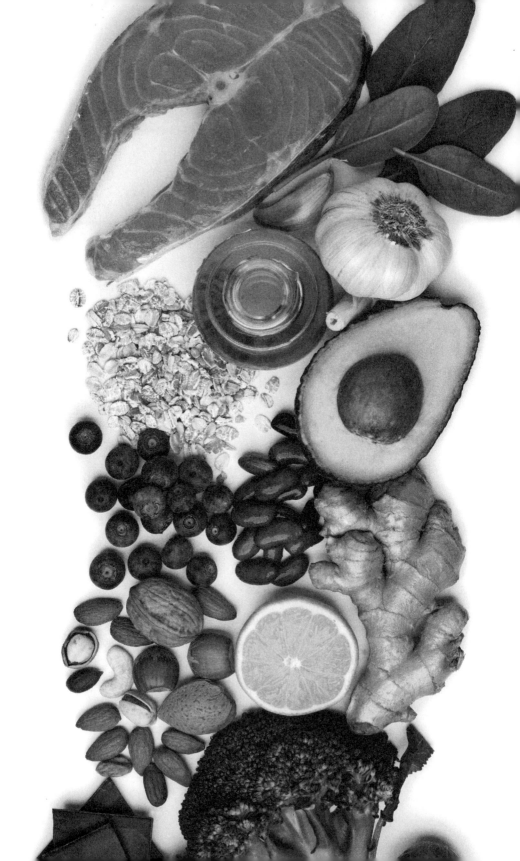

CHAPTER 5

Shopping List for Your Healthy Gut

A well-stocked pantry, refrigerator, and freezer will ensure you always have healthy options to prepare your own delicious meals. Careful shopping will help you avoid the processed and unhealthy foods that can lead to leaky gut and other digestive and health problems.

> **Note:** *Buy certified organic foods whenever possible and use pesticide- and insecticide-free products.*

Baking
- Almond meal (for *Crispy Chicken* recipe)
- Baking powder (look for "aluminum-free" on the label)
- Baking soda (aluminum-free)
- Butter (unsalted)
- Cocoa powder
- Flours (almond, amaranth, arrowroot, buckwheat, coconut, flax, millet, rice, sorghum, teff)
- Honey (raw)

- Maple syrup (dark)
- Molasses (blackstrap)
- Stevia (see page 28 for more options)
- Vanilla extract or paste

Beverages

- Amazake
- Coconut water
- Kombucha
- Sparkling water
- White wine (for *Salmon with Pecan Crust* recipe)

Breads

- Buckwheat cereal
- Rye, gluten-free
- Sprouted grain, gluten-free
- Tortillas, gluten-free corn

Canned/Bottled Goods

- Artichoke hearts (brined and oil-free)
- Beef broth/stock
- Chicken broth/stock
- Fruits (pineapple, papaya without heavy syrup)
- Olives (black, green)
- Pineapple juice (for *Beef and Vegetable Soup* recipe)
- Pumpkin
- Sockeye salmon

- Tuna fish (in water, not albacore)

Cheeses (Must be casein-free)
- Nut cheese
- Rice cheese

Condiments
- Beef and chicken broth (organic, pasture-raised)
- Dijon and yellow mustard
- Fish sauce (soy-free)
- Kimchi
- Lemon juice
- Lime juice
- Pickles
- Salsa
- Sauerkraut
- Tamari

Fresh Fruit
- Avocados
- Apples (red and green)
- Applesauce (no sugar added)
- Apricots
- Bananas
- Blackberries
- Blueberries
- Butternut squash

- Cantaloupes
- Grapes (red)
- Honeydew
- Lemons
- Limes
- Nectarines
- Oranges
- Papayas
- Peaches
- Pineapples
- Prunes
- Raspberries
- Strawberries
- Watermelon

Fresh Vegetables

- Arugula
- Asparagus
- Basil
- Broccoli
- Brussels sprouts
- Carrots (with stems, and baby carrots for snacks)
- Cauliflower
- Celery
- Chives
- Cilantro
- Garlic

- Green beans
- Kale
- Leeks
- Lettuce (spring mix, mesclun, romaine for *Creamy Coconut Balsamic Salad* recipe)
- Mushrooms (cremini/baby bella, or button)
- Onions (red, white, or yellow)
- Parsnips
- Shallots
- Spinach (baby and curly)
- Sprouts
- Squash
- Sweet potatoes
- Swiss chard
- Zucchini
- Frozen fruit
- Blackberries
- Blueberries
- Mangoes
- Peaches
- Raspberries
- Strawberries

Frozen Vegetables

- Asparagus
- Broccoli
- Corn

- Green beans
- Mixed veggies

Grains
- Arrowroot (also powder for *Creamy Chicken and Basil* recipe)
- Buckwheat
- Gluten-free oats
- Millet
- Quinoa
- Sorghum
- Teff

Herbs
- Basil (dried)
- Bay leaves (fresh)
- Oregano (fresh or dried)
- Parsley (fresh or dried)
- Sage (fresh or dried)
- Thyme (fresh or dried)

Milks (Choose your favorite)
- Almond
- Cashew (cream for *Nutty Fruit Cobbler* recipe)
- Coconut
- Hazelnut
- Hemp

- Kefir (dairy-free/low-sugar)
- Oat
- Rice

Nut/Seed Butters

- Almond butter
- Cashew butter
- Coconut butter (for *Nutty Fruit Cobbler* recipe)
- Macadamia butter
- Tahini (sesame seed butter)

Nuts/Seeds

- Almonds (raw and slivered)
- Cashews
- Hazelnuts
- Hemp seeds
- Pecans
- Pine nuts
- Pistachios
- Pumpkin seeds
- Sesame seeds
- Sunflower seeds
- Walnuts (raw)

Oils/Vinegar

- Apple cider vinegar
- Balsamic vinegar

- Coconut oil
- Flax oil
- Ghee (clarified butter)
- Olive oil (cold pressed and extra-virgin)
- Palm oil

Pasta

- Brown rice pasta
- Chickpea pasta
- Quinoa pasta
- Shirataki noodles
- Soba noodles

Proteins

Note: For meats, poultry and eggs, buy grass-fed, pasture-raised, antibiotic-/hormone-free only. For fish and seafood, fresh and wild caught from oceans and rivers is healthiest.

- Anchovy paste
- Bacon
- Beef (Get "choice" or "select" instead of "prime.")
- Chicken (fresh breasts, skinless, thin sliced)
- Eggs
- Ground beef
- Ground turkey (breast and thigh for *Turkey Meatballs* recipe)
- Halibut (Atlantic wild)
- Herring

- Lake trout (rainbow)
- Mackerel (Atlantic)
- Orange roughy
- Sardines (Pacific)
- Turkey sausage
- Wild Alaskan salmon

Rice

- Black, brown, or red
- Wild rice
- Rice alternatives
- Riced broccoli
- Riced cauliflower
- Shirataki "rice"

Snacks

- Applesauce (no added sugar)
- Dried fruit (apples, apricots, cranberries, raisins)
- Nuts (see list above)
- Yogurt (coconut, oat, or rice)

Spices

- Black pepper
- Cayenne
- Cinnamon
- Cloves (ground)
- Coriander (ground)

- Cumin
- Curry powder
- Ginger (ground)
- Italian seasoning
- Onion powder
- Sea salt (see page 31 for salt options)

Once you're done shopping, it's time to start cooking! Turn the page for the delicious, easy-to-make recipes that will get you on the road to good health.

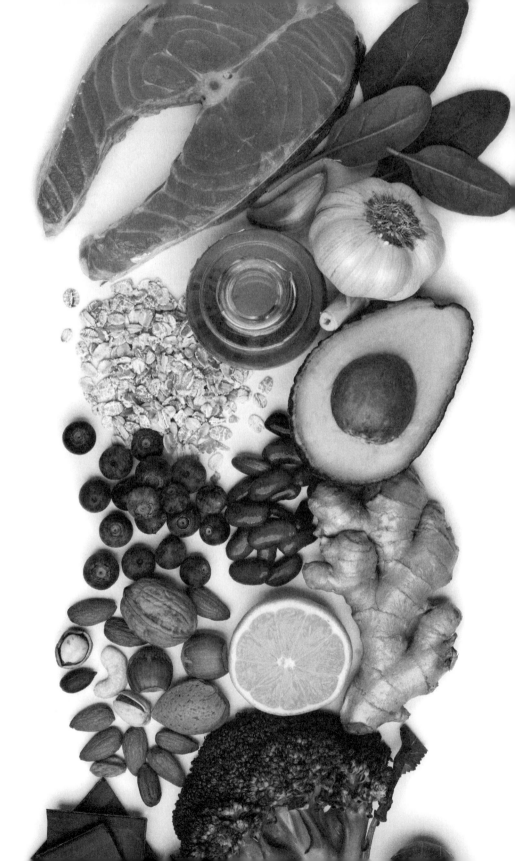

CHAPTER 6

Simply Delicious and Healthy Recipes

BREAKFASTS

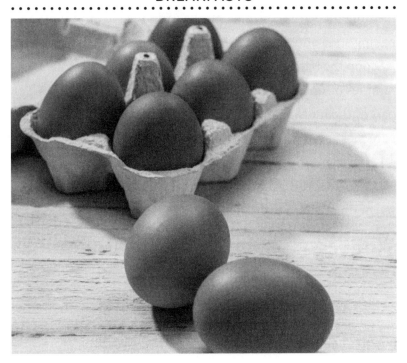

Blueberry Muffins

Servings: 12

- 3 pasture-raised eggs
- ¼ cup raw honey
- 3 tablespoons coconut oil, melted
- 1 teaspoon vanilla extract
- ¾ cup coconut flour, sifted
- 1 teaspoon baking soda
- ½ cup fresh blueberries

Preheat the oven to 325°F and line a 12-cup muffin tin with baking cups.

In a large bowl, whisk the eggs until well-blended. Whisk in the honey, coconut oil, and vanilla. Add the coconut flour and baking soda and whisk until smooth. Stir in the blueberries.

Scoop the batter into the muffin cups and bake for 20 minutes or until a toothpick inserted into the center-most part of the muffin comes out clean and warm. Let cool on a wire rack.

Leftover muffins can be refrigerated for one week. If you like, before serving leftover muffins, cut them in half and warm them by toasting them in a small pan with some coconut oil.

Crustless Veggie Quiche Cups

Servings: 9

- 1 sweet potato, cut into ½-inch cubes
- 1 tablespoon coconut oil
- 8 ounces sliced cremini mushrooms
- ¼ cup diced yellow or white onion
- 6 ounces baby spinach, chopped
- 5 pasture-raised eggs
- Pinches of sea salt and pepper

Preheat the oven to 350°F and line a 12-cup muffin tin with 9 baking cups.

Add the sweet potato to a pot of boiling water and simmer for 10 minutes; then drain well.

Melt the coconut oil in a skillet and sauté the mushroom and onion over medium heat for five minutes or until they start to soften. Add the spinach and sauté for five minutes or until it wilts and the liquid in the bottom of the pan evaporates. Set aside to cool.

Whisk together the eggs; then whisk in the cooked sweet potato and the cooled vegetable mixture. Season with sea salt and pepper; then fill the 9 muffin cups and bake for 20 minutes or until cooked through.

Leftover quiche cups can be refrigerated for four days.

· ·
LUNCHES
· ·

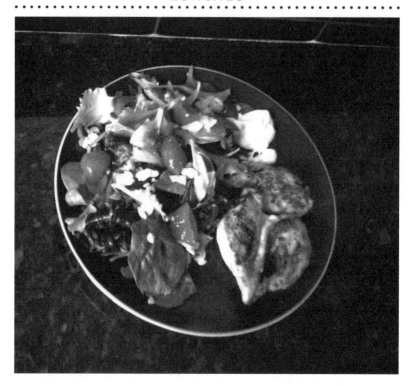

Crispy Chicken Salad
with Lemon Raspberry Vinaigrette

Servings: 4

- 1 pasture-raised egg
- 1 cup almond meal
- 1 cup coconut flour
- 1 teaspoon sea salt
- 3 pasture-raised boneless, skinless chicken breasts, cut into 1-inch thick strips
- Mixed greens (spring mix or mesclun)

Preheat the oven to 400°F and cover a baking sheet with parchment paper.

In one bowl, lightly beat the egg. Place the almond flour in another bowl and combine the coconut flour and salt in another. Dip each chicken strip in the almond flour and then the egg; then roll it in the coconut flour to coat it well.

Place the strips on the baking sheet and bake for 20 minutes or until the thickest strip is opaque and cooked through, flipping them over halfway through the bake time.

Serve the chicken strips atop the mixed greens. Dress with the lemon-raspberry vinaigrette.

Stored separately, leftover chicken and vinaigrette can each be refrigerated for four days.

Lemon-Raspberry Vinaigrette

- 1 lemon, zested and juiced
- 3 ounces fresh raspberries
- 2 tablespoons chopped shallots
- 2 cloves garlic, minced
- 1 tablespoon Dijon mustard
- ½ cup extra-virgin olive oil
- Sea salt and pepper to taste

Place all ingredients except for the oil in a small food processor and blend well. While processing, add the olive oil in a slow stream. Season to taste with salt and pepper.

Zucchini Sticks

Servings: 4

- 2 zucchinis, cut into 1-inch sticks
- 1 pasture-raised egg
- 1 tablespoon water
- ½ cup almond flour
- ½ cup coconut flour
- 2 tablespoons coconut oil, melted
- Sea salt and pepper to taste

Preheat the oven to 400°F and cover a baking sheet with parchment paper.

Sprinkle the zucchinis with salt and pepper. In one bowl, beat the egg with the water. In another bowl, mix together the almond flour and coconut flour.

Dip the zucchinis in the egg wash and then roll them in the flour mixture. Arrange them on the baking sheet so that they don't overlap.

Spoon the melted coconut oil over the zucchinis and bake for 15 to 20 minutes or until the zucchini sticks are tender and turning light brown.

Leftover zucchini sticks can be refrigerated for four days. Reheat them in a toaster oven or a skillet before serving.

Artichoke and Bacon Egg Bake

Servings: 4–6

- Coconut oil for greasing the pan
- 6 pasture-raised eggs
- 4 ounces bacon from pasture-raised hogs, cooked and chopped
- ½ cup chopped curly spinach
- ½ cup chopped brined artichoke hearts
- Half a small onion, chopped
- ⅓ cup whole coconut milk
- 1 teaspoon dried basil
- ½ teaspoon dried oregano

Preheat the oven to 300°F and grease an 8" x 8" glass pan with coconut oil.

In a large bowl, whisk the eggs until well-blended; then mix in the remaining ingredients. Pour into the greased baking dish and bake for 40 minutes or until firm and browned on top.

Leftover egg bake can be refrigerated for four days.

DINNERS/MAINS

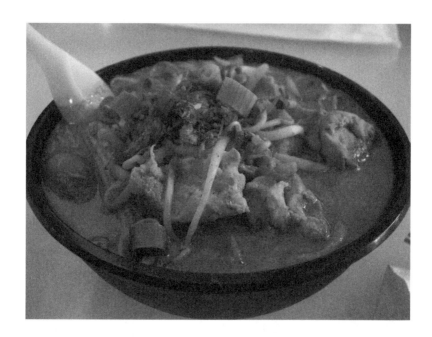

Curried Coconut-Chicken Soup

Servings: 4–6

- 1 tablespoon coconut oil
- 3 shallots, chopped
- ½ cup chopped cilantro, divided
- 4 cups pasture-raised chicken broth
- 28 ounces whole coconut milk
- 1 tablespoon raw honey
- 8 ounces cremini mushrooms, sliced
- 1 head broccoli, cut into florets
- 1 tablespoon curry powder
- 1 tablespoon fish sauce

- 1 pound pasture-raised boneless skinless chicken breast, thinly sliced
- 2 tablespoons freshly squeezed lime juice
- ¼ cup chopped green onions for garnishing
- Coconut yogurt for garnishing

Melt the coconut oil in a large pot over medium heat. Stir in the shallots and ¼ cup of the cilantro and sauté until the shallots have softened and become translucent, about five minutes.

Add the chicken broth, coconut milk, and raw honey. Bring to a simmer over medium-high heat. Stir in the mushrooms and broccoli and cook until the broccoli becomes tender, approximately five minutes. Stir in the curry powder, fish sauce, and chicken. Cook for another 10 minutes, stirring often, or until the thickest piece of chicken is opaque and cooked through.

Remove from heat and stir in the lime juice. Garnish the soup with the green onions and coconut yogurt when serving.

Leftover soup can be refrigerated for four days.

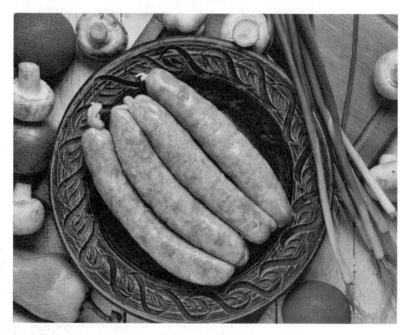

Sausage and Vegetable Bake

Servings: 4–6

- 1 pound pasture-raised turkey sausage, nitrite- and nitrate-free
- ¼ cup finely chopped celery
- ¼ cup finely chopped onion
- 2 pasture-raised eggs
- 2 cups chopped cauliflower
- ½ cup chopped yellow squash
- 1 tablespoon chopped fresh parsley
- 3 tablespoons chopped fresh sage
- 3 tablespoons chopped fresh thyme
- 1 garlic clove, grated

- ¼ teaspoon sea salt
- ⅛ teaspoon black pepper

Preheat the oven to 350°F and grease an 8" x 8" glass pan.

If necessary, remove the casing from sausage and break the meat into small bits. Place the sausage in a large skillet over medium heat. Add the celery and onion and cook for about 10 minutes, stirring often, or until the veggies are soft and the sausage is completely cooked.

Meanwhile, in a large bowl, lightly beat the eggs. Add the cooked sausage mixture to the bowl; then add the remaining ingredients. Whisk until well-blended.

Pour the mixture into the baking dish and cover it tightly with foil. Bake for 30 minutes, then uncover the bake and continue baking it for 5 to 10 minutes or until the edges start to brown.

Leftover bake can be refrigerated for four days.

Note: You can vary this recipe by using pork sausage in place of the turkey sausage.

Beef and Vegetable Stew

Servings: 4–6

- 1 pound grass-fed ground beef
- 2 cloves garlic, minced
- 1 medium onion, chopped
- 1 stalk celery, diced
- 1 cup grass-fed beef broth
- ¼ cup pineapple juice
- 1 teaspoon dried parsley
- 1 teaspoon dried thyme
- 1 cup chopped carrots
- 1 sweet potato, cubed
- 1 parsnip, peeled and cubed
- 2 bay leaves
- 1 tablespoon coconut flour

Place the beef in a large pot over medium-high heat. Cook, stirring often, for about three minutes or until the beef has started to brown. Stir in the garlic, onion, and celery and sauté for four minutes. Turn the heat down to medium and pour in the broth and juice. Add the herbs, carrots, sweet potato, parsnip, and bay leaves, and stir to combine.

Cover and simmer over medium heat until the carrots, sweet potato, and parsnips are softening, about 15 minutes. Uncover and stir in the coconut flour; then cook for an additional five minutes. Remove the bay leaves before serving.

Leftover soup can be refrigerated for four days.

Note: *You can vary this recipe by using ground lamb in place of the ground beef.*

Vegetable Rice Stir-Fry

Servings: 4

- 2 tablespoons coconut oil
- ½ cup chopped onion
- 1 teaspoon ground ginger
- 2 cloves garlic, chopped
- 2 cups diced butternut squash
- 4 carrots, chopped
- 1 zucchini, chopped
- 1 head kale, chopped
- 1 cup slivered almonds
- 2 cups cooked cauliflower rice

Melt the oil in a large skillet over medium heat. Stir in the onion, ginger, and garlic and sauté for three to five minutes or until tender. Add the rest of the vegetables and cover. Cook, covered, for five minutes; then uncover the skillet and continue cooking for another two to three minutes, stirring often. Stir the almonds and cooked cauliflower rice into the vegetables and serve warm.

Leftover stir-fry can be refrigerated for four days.

Note: For more crunch, toast the almonds in a dry skillet for three to four minutes over medium heat or until the almonds are light brown; then stir them into the stir-fry.

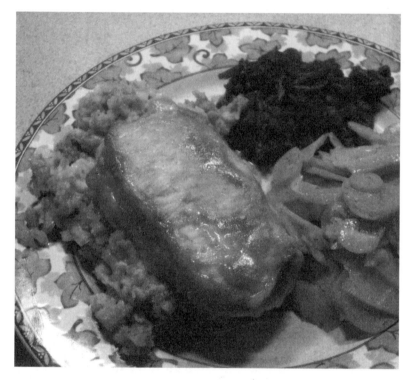

Honey Mustard Pork with Jicama and Green Apples

Servings: 4

FOR THE PORK

- 2 tablespoons coconut oil
- 1 pound pork tenderloin from pasture-raised hogs, cut into ½-inch thick slices
- 1 head of green or red leaf lettuce
- 1 green apple
- 1 jicama, peeled and cut into matchsticks
- 2 pasture-raised hard-boiled eggs, chopped

FOR THE DRESSING
- ¼ cup freshly squeezed lemon juice
- 2 tablespoons Dijon mustard
- 2 tablespoons raw honey
- 1 clove garlic, minced
- ½ cup extra-virgin olive oil

Melt the oil in a large skillet over medium heat; then stir in the pork. Sauté for three minutes; then flip over each piece. Cook for another three minutes or until the thickest piece of pork is opaque when cut in half.

Remove the pork to a plate and let cool; then cut into bite-sized pieces. While the pork cools, make the dressing by combining the lemon juice, mustard, honey, and garlic in a food processor. While processing, add the olive oil in a slow stream.

Chop the lettuce and apple; then toss with the cooked pork, jicama, and eggs. Add the dressing and toss well again before serving.

Leftover dressed salad can be refrigerated for one day. If stored separately, the pork can be refrigerated for two days and the dressing for four days.

Note: *Jicama is a fiber-rich Mexican turnip.*

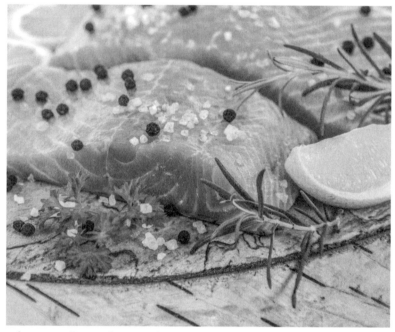

Pineapple Salsa Salmon

Servings: 4

- 1 tablespoon coconut oil, melted
- Juice of half a lemon
- 2 cloves garlic, minced
- 1 pound wild salmon

Preheat the oven to 350°F and grease a glass 8" x 8" baking pan. Combine the coconut oil, lemon, and garlic in small bowl. Coat the salmon with the mixture and bake for 20 minutes or until the center of the salmon flakes cleanly apart. To serve, top the salmon with the pineapple salsa.

Leftover salmon can be refrigerated for two days.

Pineapple Salsa

- 2 teaspoons coconut oil
- 3 cups diced pineapple
- 1½ cups chopped onion
- 1 green apple, diced
- 2 cloves garlic, minced
- ½ cup pineapple juice
- 2 tablespoons apple cider vinegar
- ½ cup cilantro or parsley, finely chopped
- 2 tablespoons freshly squeezed lime juice
- ½ teaspoon sea salt

Melt the oil in a large skillet over medium-high heat. Add the pineapple and onion and cook for one minute or until lightly browned. Add the apple and garlic and sauté for another minute. Stir in the pineapple juice and vinegar and cook for six minutes, stirring occasionally. Remove from the heat and stir in the remaining ingredients.

Serve warm over the salmon or refrigerate and serve cool as a salsa dip. Leftover salsa can be refrigerated for four days.

Salmon with Pecan Crust

Servings: 4–6

- 2 tablespoons finely chopped fresh basil leaves
- 1½ tablespoons Dijon mustard
- ¼ teaspoon kosher salt
- 1/8 teaspoon black pepper
- 2 ounces dry white wine
- 2 tablespoons freshly squeezed lemon juice
- 1 pound wild salmon
- 2 tablespoons extra-virgin olive oil
- ½ cup chopped pecans

Preheat the oven to 400°F and get out a glass 9" x 13" baking pan.

In a small bowl, mix together the basil, mustard, salt, pepper, white wine, and lemon juice. Coat the salmon well with the basil mixture and arrange the salmon in the baking dish, leaving enough room between the pieces so that they all bake evenly.

Mix the olive oil and pecans together, then spoon even amounts of the mixture over each piece of salmon.

Bake the salmon for 15 to 20 minutes or until the center flakes apart cleanly. Serve with your choice of vegetables.

Leftover salmon can be refrigerated for two days.

Creamy Chicken and Basil

Servings: 4

- 2 tablespoons coconut oil
- 4 free-range boneless, skinless chicken breasts, cut into evenly sized large pieces
- 1¼ cups whole coconut milk
- 1 teaspoon sea salt
- 1 teaspoon freshly ground black pepper
- 2 tablespoons fresh basil, chopped finely
- 1 cup pasture-raised chicken broth
- 2 tablespoons arrowroot powder
- 1 cup curly spinach, chopped

Melt the oil in a large skillet over medium heat; then stir in the chicken. Sauté for about five minutes per side until the chicken is almost fully cooked. Remove the chicken to a plate.

Meanwhile, whisk together the coconut milk, salt, pepper, and basil. In another bowl, whisk the broth with the arrowroot until the arrowroot has dissolved.

Pour the coconut mixture into the skillet and bring it to just under a boil. Slowly whisk the broth mixture into the coconut mixture until it thickens. Nestle the chicken back into the skillet and add the spinach. Cover and let gently simmer until the spinach has softened and the thickest piece of chicken is opaque and cooked through, about five minutes.

Leftover chicken can be refrigerated for two days.

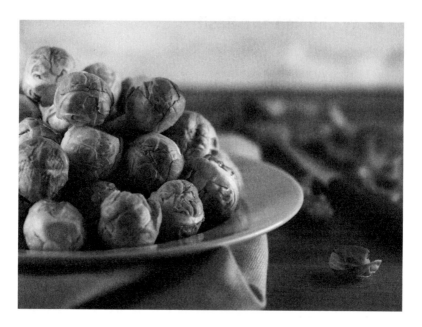

Creamy Coconut Balsamic Salad with Brussels Sprouts, Walnuts, and Cranberries

Servings: 4

FOR THE SALAD

- 8 ounces Brussels sprouts, trimmed and halved
- Coconut oil for roasting
- 1 head romaine lettuce, washed and chopped
- 1 cup raw walnuts, chopped
- ½ cup unsweetened dried cranberries

FOR THE DRESSING

- 2 tablespoons whole coconut milk
- 1 tablespoon aged balsamic vinegar

- 1 teaspoon apple cider vinegar or freshly squeezed lemon juice
- 1 teaspoon Dijon mustard
- ½ teaspoon dried basil
- ¼ teaspoon sea salt
- ¼ cup extra-virgin olive oil

Preheat the oven to 375°F and cover a baking sheet with parchment paper.

In a medium bowl, toss the sprouts with the coconut oil, coating them well. Arrange them on the baking sheet; then bake for 15 to 20 minutes or until they're turning light brown. While the sprouts are roasting, make the dressing by combining the coconut milk, vinegars, mustard, basil, and salt in a food processor. While processing, add the olive oil in a slow stream.

Toss the roasted Brussels sprouts with the lettuce, walnuts, and cranberries. Add the dressing and toss again before serving.

Stored separately, leftover sprouts and dressing can each be refrigerated for four days.

SIDES

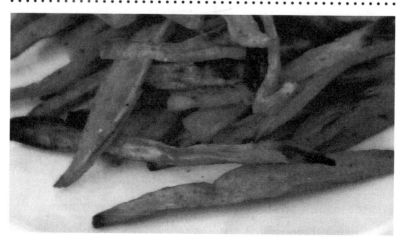

Sweet Potato Fries

Servings: 4

- 2 large sweet potatoes, unpeeled, sliced into ½-inch thick strips
- 2 tablespoons coconut oil, melted
- 2 teaspoons sea salt

Preheat the oven to 300°F. In a large bowl, coat the sweet potato strips with the oil, then sprinkle with salt. Arrange the sweet potatoes on a parchment-covered baking sheet, using two sheets if necessary to prevent the strips from overlapping. Bake for 20 minutes or until golden brown, flipping halfway through.

Serve with Yogurt Ranch Vegetable Dip on 99.

Leftover fries can be refrigerated for four days. Reheat them in a toaster oven or in a skillet before serving.

Lemon Tahini Kale Salad

Servings: 4

- 1½ tablespoons tahini
- 2 tablespoons extra-virgin olive oil
- Juice of 1 lemon
- 2 teaspoons apple cider vinegar
- ½ teaspoon anchovy paste
- 1 bunch kale

Combine all ingredients except for the kale in a food processor and blend until smooth. Steam the kale and chop or tear it into pieces. Pour the lemon tahini sauce over the kale and toss well before serving.

Leftover sauce and kale can be refrigerated for one day together or for three days if kept separately.

Note: *The sauce also makes a great salad dressing!*

FAMILY/COMFORT FOOD

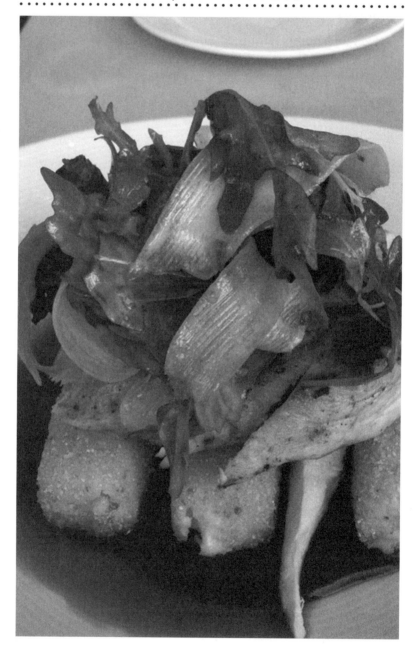

Chicken Fingers

Servings: 4

- 1 cup almond meal
- 2 teaspoons Italian seasoning
- 2 teaspoons garlic powder
- 1 teaspoon sea salt
- 1 teaspoon pepper
- 2 pasture-raised eggs
- 1 pound pasture-raised boneless, skinless chicken breasts or thighs, cut into 1-inch strips

Preheat the oven to 375°F and cover a baking sheet with parchment paper.

In one bowl, combine the almond meal, seasonings, salt, and pepper. In another bowl, lightly beat the eggs. Dip the chicken strips into the beaten egg and then roll in the almond mixture until coated.

Arrange strips on the baking sheet and bake for 20 to 30 minutes or until cooked through, flipping them over halfway through the bake time. Serve with Yogurt Ranch Dip on page 99.

Leftover chicken can be refrigerated for four days.

Super Sloppy Joes

Servings: 4–6

- 1 pound grass-fed ground beef
- 1 small onion, chopped
- ½ cup mashed canned pumpkin
- ½ cup grass-fed beef broth
- 1 tablespoon apple cider vinegar
- 2 teaspoons cumin
- 2 teaspoons yellow mustard
- 1 tablespoon blackstrap molasses
- 2 teaspoons anchovy paste
- ½ teaspoon sea salt
- Dash of ground cloves
- Dash of ground ginger

Brown the meat and onions in a large skillet over medium-high heat for about five minutes, stirring often. Drain the meat mixture and put it back in the skillet. Add the rest of the ingredients and mix well. Simmer for 20 minutes, covered, over low heat.

Serve with Sweet Potato Fries on page 92.

Leftover Sloppy Joes can be refrigerated for four days.

Taco Salad

Servings: 4

- 1 pound pasture-raised ground turkey (or grass-fed ground beef)
- 2 tablespoons mashed papaya
- 1½ teaspoons ground cumin
- 1 teaspoon dried oregano
- ½ teaspoon ground coriander
- ¼ teaspoon garlic powder
- ¼ teaspoon onion powder
- 1 teaspoon sea salt
- ½ teaspoon black pepper
- ½ cup free-range chicken broth
- 2 tablespoons apple cider vinegar

TOPPINGS:

- Shredded lettuce
- Chopped black olives
- Coconut yogurt
- Chopped cilantro leaves
- Pineapple Salsa (see page 87)
- Guacamole (see page 98)

Brown the turkey in a large skillet over medium-high heat for about five minutes, stirring often. Drain the meat and put it back in skillet. Stir in the papaya, all the spices, and the broth and vinegar. Simmer for about 15 minutes, stirring occasionally. Serve with your choice of toppings.

Leftover taco salad without toppings can be refrigerated for four days.

SNACKS

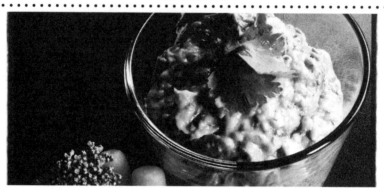

Guacamole Dip

Servings: 4–6

- 2 ripe avocados
- 2 tablespoons freshly squeezed lemon juice
- ¼ cup chopped onion
- 2 small garlic cloves, minced
- ½ teaspoon sea salt or more to taste
- Handful of chopped cilantro leaves (optional)
- Veggies for serving

Scoop avocados out of their shells and mash them in a bowl. Add remaining ingredients and mix well. Serve with fresh chopped carrots, celery, broccoli, jicama, or other vegetables you enjoy.

Leftover guacamole can be refrigerated for two days. Carefully cover the top of the guacamole with plastic wrap to prevent air from coming into contact with it. (Contact with air will make the guacamole turn brown.)

Yogurt Ranch Vegetable Dip

Servings: About 1 cup

- 1 cup coconut yogurt
- 1 teaspoon dried dill
- ½ teaspoon onion powder
- ½ teaspoon garlic powder
- ½ teaspoon dried parsley
- Sea salt and pepper to taste
- Veggies for serving

Mix ingredients until well blended, then add salt and pepper to taste. Serve with fresh chopped carrots, celery, broccoli, jicama, or other vegetables you enjoy.

Leftover dip can be refrigerated for four days.

Creamy Deviled Eggs

Servings: 12 egg halves

- 6 pasture-raised hard-boiled eggs
- ½ cup coconut yogurt
- 1 green onion, green part only, minced
- 1 tablespoon dried sage
- 2 teaspoons Dijon mustard
- ½ teaspoon sea salt

Carefully cut each egg in half and tip out the yolk into a medium mixing bowl. Mash yolks with a fork and then stir in the remaining ingredients until the mixture is smooth. With a regular teaspoon, scoop the filling into each egg white half, mounding the filling into a small hill. You can help the halved eggs stay balanced by placing the filling all along the length of the egg white half rather than just in the indentation left by the departed egg yolk.

Set the eggs into a rimmed dish (or better yet, in a long and narrow serving dish) so that they don't tip over or scoot themselves onto the floor. You can either serve immediately or cover them and keep them into the fridge for later.

Leftover eggs can be refrigerated for four days.

Pistachio and Hemp Seed Trail Mix

Servings: About 2 cups

- ¼ cup shelled pistachios
- ½ cup hemp seeds (also called hemp hearts)
- ¼ cup halved pecans
- ¼ cup unsweetened raisins or dried cranberries
- ¼ cup unsweetened dried cherries
- Chopped 70% dark chocolate (optional)
- Unsweetened coconut flakes (optional)

Place all ingredients in a sealed bag and shake well.

Trail mix can be stored in an airtight container at room temperature for two weeks or refrigerated for one month. If the temperature is higher than 75°F, however, the chocolate may melt.

> **Note:** *You can vary this recipe by substituting walnuts or macadamia nuts for the pistachios and pecans or other dried fruits in place of the raisins and cherries. Just be sure to choose unsweetened dried fruits!*

Easy Delicious Bread

Servings: 2 loaves of 10–12 slices each

- Coconut oil for greasing
- 2 cups blanched almond flour
- ½ teaspoon sea salt
- 1 teaspoon baking soda
- 3 pasture-raised eggs
- ¼ cup raw honey
- 2 teaspoons sparkling water

Preheat the oven to 300°F and thoroughly grease two small loaf pans (approximately 6" x 3" each) with coconut oil.

In one bowl, mix together the almond flour, sea salt, and baking soda. In another bowl, whisk the eggs, then whisk in the raw honey and sparkling water. Stir the wet ingredients into the dry ingredients.

Scoop the batter into the loaf pans and bake for 35 to 45 minutes or until a toothpick inserted in the middle comes out clean. Let cool before slicing.

Completely cooled bread can be stored in an airtight container for four days at room temperature or refrigerated for one week.

Avocado, Almond, and Fruit Smoothie

Servings: 2

- 1 avocado
- 1 cup frozen mangoes
- ½ cup frozen strawberries or peaches
- 2 tablespoons raw almond butter
- ½ cup water
- ½ cup whole coconut milk or coconut yogurt

Add all ingredients to the blender. Blend until smooth and serve. This is best enjoyed immediately.

Coconut Mango Smoothie

Servings: 2

- 1 cup frozen mangoes
- ½ banana, fresh or frozen
- ½ cup whole coconut milk
- ½ cup water
- 1 teaspoon raw honey

Add all ingredients to blender. Blend until smooth and serve. This is best enjoyed immediately.

DESSERTS

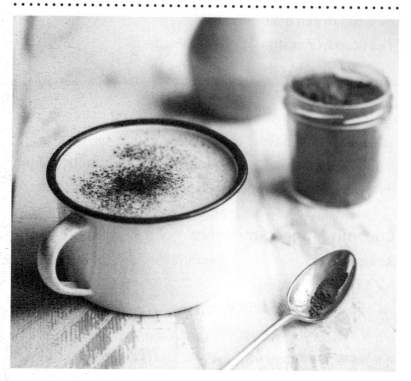

Healthy Hot Chocolate

Servings: 1

- 1 cup unsweetened almond milk
- 2 tablespoons raw cacao powder
- Maple syrup to taste

Pour the milk into a small pan and warm over medium heat. Whisk in the cacao powder and sweeten to taste with the maple syrup. Serve immediately.

Coconut Cacao Bites

Servings: 12

- ⅓ cup raw honey
- 2 tablespoons coconut oil
- 3 tablespoons raw cacao powder
- ½ teaspoon ground cinnamon
- ¼ cup almond butter
- ¼ cup unsweetened flaked coconut
- ¼ cup coconut flour
- 1 teaspoon vanilla paste (or extract)

Cover a baking sheet or a tray with parchment or wax paper.

In a small saucepan over medium heat, combine the honey, coconut oil, cacao powder, and cinnamon. Stir continuously for several minutes until you have a chocolate syrup-like texture.

Remove from the heat and add the remaining ingredients. Stir until completely combined, then drop by the spoonful on the covered sheet or tray. Chill for approximately 45 minutes or until firm and chewy.

Cocoa bites can be refrigerated for one week.

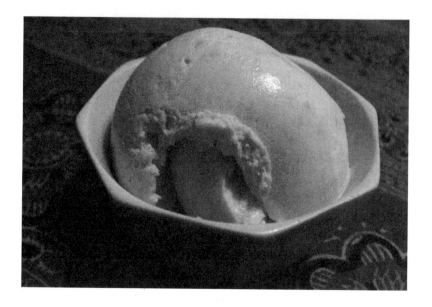

Peach Coconut Milk Ice Cream

Servings: 4 cups

- 2 cups whole coconut milk
- 2 cups frozen sliced peaches
- ½ cup maple syrup
- 2 teaspoons vanilla paste (or extract)
- Pinch of sea salt

Handful of chopped toasted nuts for garnishing (optional)

Put all ingredients except for the nuts in a blender and blend until smooth. Pour into an ice cream machine and freeze according to the machine's instructions. If you like, serve garnished with toasted nuts.

Nutty Fruit Cobbler with Cashew Cream

Servings: 6

- 3 cups fresh or frozen and thawed blueberries (or other fruit)
- ¼ cup freshly squeezed lemon juice
- ⅔ cup coconut palm sugar
- 1½ cups raw pecans or other raw nuts
- ¾ teaspoon ground cinnamon
- 1 dash sea salt
- ½ cup coconut butter, chopped into 8 pieces
- 1 recipe Whipped Cashew Cream

Preheat the oven to 350°F and thoroughly grease an 8" x 8" baking dish.

Place the berries in the baking dish and drizzle on the lemon juice. In a food processor, combine the coconut palm sugar, nuts, cinnamon, and salt. Add the coconut butter pieces and pulse until the mixture resembles coarse crumbs.

Sprinkle the nut mixture over berries and bake for 20 to 25 minutes or until the topping is golden brown and berries are tender. Serve with Whipped Cashew Cream.

Cobbler can be stored at room temperature for two days or refrigerated for one week.

Whipped Cashew Cream

- 1 cup raw cashews
- 1¼ cups filtered warm water, divided
- ½ teaspoon sea salt
- 1 teaspoon vanilla paste (or extract)
- 1 teaspoon raw honey

Combine the cashews, one cup filtered water, and sea salt. Let soak for six hours. Drain the cashews and transfer to a blender. Add the rest of the filtered water and the remaining ingredients. Blend until you have a smooth mixture that resembles whipped cream; then serve.

Cashew cream can be refrigerated for four days.

Measurement Conversions

Volume Equivalents (Liquid)

US Standard	US Standard (ounces)	Metric (approximate)
2 tablespoons	1 fl. oz.	20 mL
¼ cup	2 fl. oz.	60 mL
½ cup	4 fl. oz.	120 mL
1 cup	8 fl. oz.	240 mL
1 ½ cups	12 fl. oz.	355 mL
2 cups or 1 pint	16 fl. oz.	475 mL
4 cups or 1 quart	32 fl. oz.	1 L
1 gallon	128 fl. oz.	4 L

Volume Equivalents (Dry)

US Standard	Metric (approximate)
⅛ teaspoon	0.5 mL
¼ teaspoon	1 mL
½ teaspoon	2 mL
¾ teaspoon	4 mL
1 teaspoon	5 mL
1 tablespoon	15 mL
¼ cup	59 mL
⅓ cup	79 mL
½ cup	118 mL
⅔ cup	156 mL
¾ cup	177 mL
1 cup	235 mL
2 cups or 1 pint	475 mL
3 cups	700 mL
4 cups or 1 quart	1 L

Weight Equivalents

US Standard	Metric (approximate)
1/2 ounce	15 g
1 ounce	30 g
2 ounces	60 g
4 ounces	115 g
8 ounces	225 g
12 ounces	340 g
16 ounces or 1 pound	455 g

Oven Temperatures

Fahrenheit	Celsius (approximate)
250°F	120°C
300°F	150°C
325°F	165°C
350°F	180°C
375°F	190°C
400°F	200°C
425°F	220°C
450°F	230°C

PART 2

How to Keep on Track

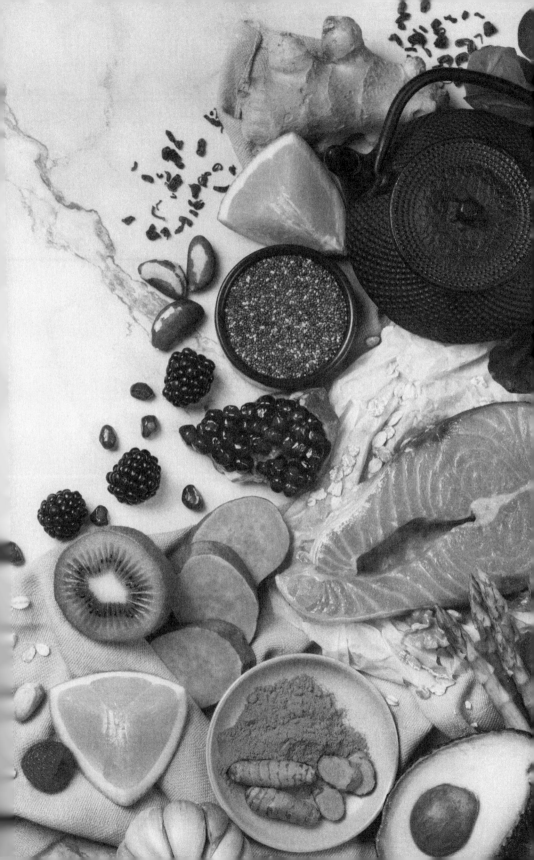

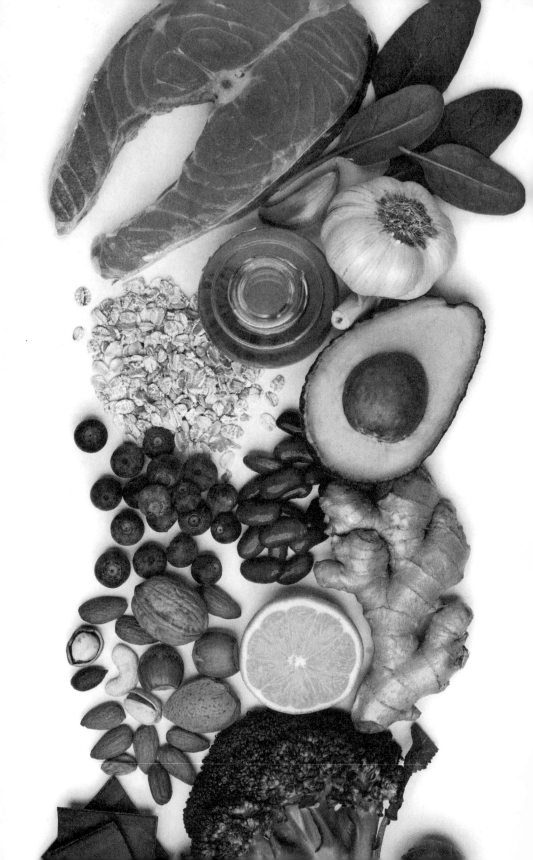

CHAPTER 7

The Skinny on Fats

Fat has gotten a bad rap due in part to many health organizations and some misinformed media that once touted low-fat diets as the standard for good health. The truth is that our bodies rely on the presence of fat. Some vitamins, such as A, D, E, and K, can only be absorbed into our bloodstream in the presence of fat. Dietary fat, also known as fatty acids, is found in foods from both plants and animals. Fat adds flavor to the food we eat and satisfies our hunger. That said, the excess calories from eating too much fat of any type can lead to weight gain. Foods contain a mixture of fatty acids, but the predominant type of fat they contain determines whether or not they are healthy. I will explain the difference.

Bad Fat

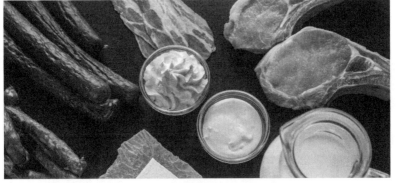

You've probably heard the term "trans fat," which is short for "trans fatty acids." Trans fat appears in packaged foods that contain partially hydrogenated (hai DRAA juh nay tuhd) vegetable oils. These are the worst kinds of fats. Trans fat can raise your LDL ("bad") cholesterol. At the same time, trans fat can suppress HDL ("good") cholesterol levels. Research has also linked trans fats to an increased risk of inflammation in the body. Inflammation can cause harmful health effects, including heart disease, diabetes, and stroke. Trans fats and fat from conventionally raised meat sources are potentially harmful to your health. Trans fats can be found in the following foods:

- Bacon
- Biscuits
- Butter, ghee, suet, lard, coconut oil, and palm oil
- Cakes
- Cheese
- Chocolate and chocolate spreads
- Coconut milk and coconut cream
- Cream, crème fraîche, and sour cream
- Cured meats like salami, chorizo, and pancetta
- Fatty cuts of meat
- Ice cream
- Margarine (stick and tub)
- Milkshakes
- Pastries, such as pies, quiches, and croissants
- Sausages, sausage rolls
- Vegetable shortening

Don't worry because all the foods listed above can be raised to have or can be made with healthy, non-trans fats.

> **GO WITH YOUR GUT TIP**
> ### Read the Label
> Labeling laws allow food companies to round down to zero and claim "no trans fats" or "zero grams of trans fats" if the amount per serving is less than 0.5 grams. However, the product still contains hydrogenated oils. As always, ignore the front-of-package marketing hype and read the ingredient list carefully. See more about *How to Decipher Labels* on page 147.

Good Fats

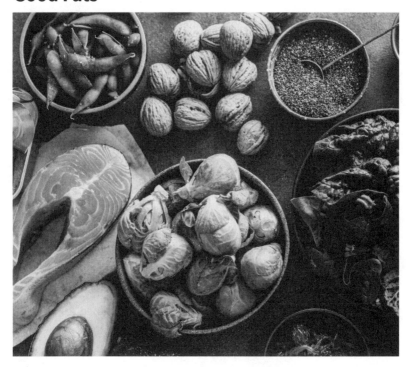

Monounsaturated fat and polyunsaturated fat are considered "heart-healthy" fats and are better choices for your diet. Saturated fat (found in animal products) can be a healthy source of fats if the food source it comes from has been grown or raised in an organic setting.

Monounsaturated Fats

These good fats are present in a variety of foods and oils. Research has consistently shown that eating foods that contain monounsaturated fat can improve your blood cholesterol level and decrease your risk for cardiovascular disease. These foods include:

- Avocado
- Nuts (almonds, cashews, peanuts, pecans)
- Olive oil and peanut oil
- Peanut butter and almond butter

Polyunsaturated Fats

Polyunsaturated fats are known as "essential fats" because the body cannot make them and we need to get them from foods. Plant-based foods and oils are the primary sources of this fat. In the same way that monounsaturated fats can decrease your risk for heart disease, omega-3 fatty acids, a type of polyunsaturated fat, have been shown to be particularly beneficial for the heart. Omega-3s may not only decrease the risk of coronary artery disease, but they also help to lower blood pressure levels and guard against irregular heart rates. The following foods contain omega-3 fatty acids:

- Chia seeds
- Fish oils
- Flaxseed
- Herring
- Salmon
- Sardines
- Trout
- Tuna
- Walnuts

Along with omega-3 fatty acids, omega-6 fatty acids play a crucial role in brain function. As a type of polyunsaturated fatty acid (PUFA), omega-6 helps stimulate skin and hair growth, maintain bone health, regulate metabolism, and maintain the reproductive system. The following foods contain omega-6 fatty acids:

- Free-range animal products
- Seeds (pumpkin seeds, sunflower seeds, sesame seeds)
- Vegetable oils (corn oil, safflower oil, sesame oil, sunflower oil)
- Walnuts

GO WITH YOUR GUT TIP

All Oils Aren't Equal

Certain polyunsaturated fats (e.g., vegetable oils such as soy, corn, canola, and cottonseed) contain high amounts of omega-6 fatty acids and lack the balancing effects of omega-3 fatty acids. These oils have been shown to depress the immune system over time. Many of them also contain harmful free radicals because they are refined under high heat and pressure. In general, vegetable oil is a refined blend of neutral oils that is high in pro-inflammatory fats and lacks micronutrients. Olive oil is made from pressed olives, and extra-virgin versions of olive oil are the least processed and retain the most beneficial compounds. Olive oil, while healthy, cannot be heated to high temperatures because it will lose its beneficial qualities.

How to Buy Healthy Oils

1. Do not buy oil in a clear container. The container must shield the oil from light, as light damages healthy oils.

2. Check the expiration date on the container. Nutrients have a shelf life. Think of it this way: If there are no nutrients in the oil, it can last forever.

3. Look for expeller or cold-pressed oils found mostly at health-food and high-end stores. Avoid oils processed at high temperature or under high pressure. Hydrogenation destroys valuable nutrients and creates toxins.

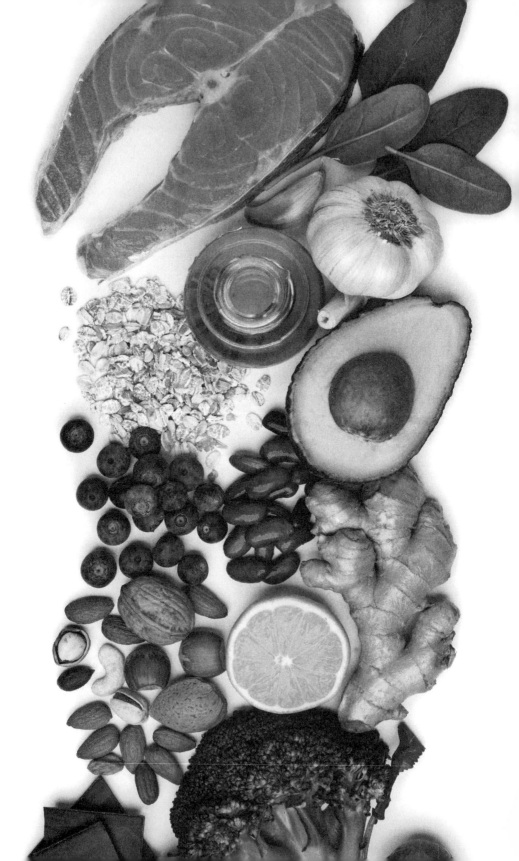

CHAPTER 8

Your Restaurant CHEAT Sheet

Everyone needs a break from making meals and doing the dishes once in a while. But how do you stick to your Heal Your Leaky Gut Diet when you're not the one preparing the food? Here are some tips to remember when eating out:

- Look at the restaurant's menu online before you go. Decide which gut-friendly dishes you're going to get ahead of time so that you're not tempted by unhealthy options once you're there. It's also a good idea to call ahead to make sure you will be able to order to suit your needs.
- Pass on the bread basket. (Most are loaded with wheat flour and gluten.)
- Bring your own sea salt and stevia for seasoning and sweetening, respectively. (Always taste first before you add seasoning.)
- When eating out for breakfast, request a salad, veggies, or fruit instead of the hash browns, home fries, or processed grits. If eating at a diner, stay away from the table maple

syrup. Ask for pure maple syrup instead—the darker kind has more minerals and antioxidants. (You might have to pay a bit more, but it's worth it!)

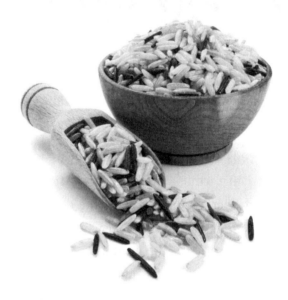

- Get wild rice instead of white rice.
- Request sauces and dressing on the side so that you can control how much you add to your dish.
- Ask for nuts on your salads instead of croutons.
- Skip dessert and have an espresso or American coffee instead. If you want to splurge, share a dessert with your dining companion. Take a few bites and leave the rest or take leftovers home for another time.
- Avoid anything on the menu described as *Alfredo, blackened, breaded, creamed, crispy, dipped, fried, marbled,* or *scalloped.* These are red flags for fat, refined salt, and

oxidized oils (oils from unsaturated fats cooked at high temperatures). Choose healthier options described as *baked, broiled, grilled, roasted, seared,* or *steamed.*

- If you're an omnivore, meat that comes from grass-fed animals raised at a family (not factory) farm is a perfectly healthy choice. The leaner cuts of beef include flank steak, skirt steak, tenderloin, sirloin, or filet mignon. A rib eye is the fattiest of all steaks; an 8-ounce rib eye steak has approximately 41.6 grams of fat.

- Chicken is another good protein, when pasture raised. Breast meat is best.

- Ask questions. Don't be afraid to ask your server how a dish is prepared. Chefs are trained to use lots of butter and salt because they make food taste good. If a dish you're eyeing is prepared with lots of butter and oil, ask if the chef might be able to prepare it differently, or choose something else. Many restaurants are aware of and can accommodate food allergies and dietary preferences these days.

- Aperitifs (pre-dinner drinks) are meant to stimulate the appetite, and digestifs (after-dinner drinks) are for aiding digestion. I recommend avoiding both. Have a seltzer with lime or lemon instead. Cocktails such as margaritas, piña coladas, and other mixed drinks are high in sugar, and dessert wines (e.g., port or muscat) have up to 7 grams of sugar per serving.

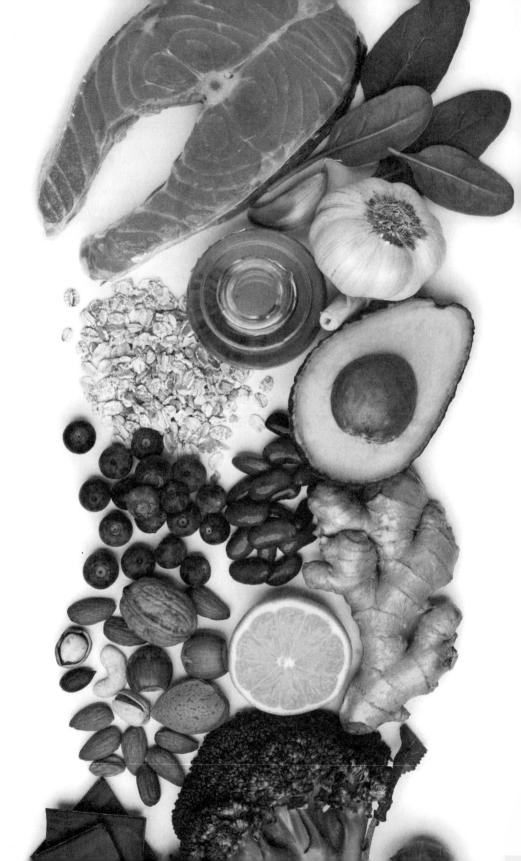

CHAPTER 9

Natural Remedies and Supplements for LGS

While changing your diet and lifestyle are the best ways to treat a leaky gut, some herbs and supplements help treat LGS and the conditions it causes. Here are some remedies I recommend to my patients:

Herbs

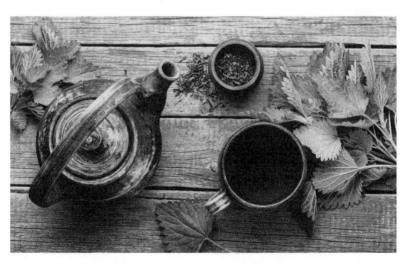

- **Aloe vera.** Often sold as a juice, aloe vera is thought to treat symptoms of diarrhea and constipation. The anti-inflammatory properties of aloe vera are thought to reduce inflammation in the gut. Taking aloe vera (2–4 tablespoons four times a day) can soothe the esophagus and help it heal from acid reflux and gastroesophageal reflux disease (GERD). Aloe vera is best taken before meals or on an empty stomach.
- **Berry leaves.** Teas made from blueberry, blackberry, or raspberry contain tannins, which may decrease inflammation and reduce symptoms of diarrhea.
- **Chamomile.** This daisy-like plant can be consumed in tea and as a liquid or capsule. One small study found that chamomile reduced spasms in the gut causing pain.
- **Ginger.** This root plant may reduce gas and bloating. The active ingredient, gingerol, has antibacterial, anti-nausea, and sedative properties that may reduce pain and restore gut function.
- **Licorice root.** This powerhouse ingredient is able to help control *H. pylori*, the detrimental bacteria that can enter your body through your digestive tract and cause inflammation. Licorice root can also improve irritation and cuts in the mucosal lining of the esophagus and stomach. People with high blood pressure, congestive heart failure, kidney disease, low potassium levels, and pregnancy should avoid licorice products. Licorice should be taken under the guidance of your doctor.

- **Peppermint oil.** Peppermint is the first herb to be approved by the American College of Gastroenterology for treating irritable bowel syndrome (IBS). Peppermint is thought to relax the muscles of the gut to improve motility (the passage of food through the gut). Studies show that the herb is even more effective than antispasmodic medication.
- **Slippery elm.** In powdered form, this herb can soothe heartburn and mild stomach discomfort. It has been shown to relieve constipation in people with IBS-C (IBS with constipation), according to one study.
- **Triphala.** Triphala is made from the fruit of the amalaki tree and contains powerful anti-inflammatory compounds that may help reduce constipation, abdominal pain, and bloating.

Supplements

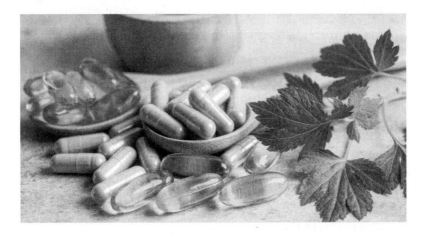

Research has shown the following supplements to have promising results in the treatment of leaky gut syndrome. As always, consult with your doctor before taking any new medication:

- **Berberine.** Berberine is a bioactive plant-based compound that may be beneficial as a leaky gut supplement. It has antioxidant, anti-inflammatory, antibacterial, and antiviral properties. Berberine is typically used to treat inflammatory bowel diseases.

- **Butyrate.** Butyrate is a short chain fatty acid that provides fuel for cells lining the gut. In fact, it provides the major energy source for the cells of the gut lining. Butyrate has anti-inflammatory effects in the gut by suppressing certain inflammatory cells. It also supports healthy gut bacteria and helps regulate natural movement in the gut. Research suggests that butyrate supplementation may stimulate mucus production and help tighten the junctions in the lining of the tract.

- **Collagen peptides.** Collagen is an important protein found in almost every tissue of the body. Better known for its effects on the skin, it may also play a beneficial role in gut health. Collagen peptides are the most easily digestible form of collagen. A recent study found that collagen peptides prevented further breakdown of the intestinal lining. In an earlier study in 2012, the use of gelatin tannate, a supplement containing naturally occurring collagen, demonstrated anti-inflammatory properties in the gut.

- **Curcumin.** Curcumin is the plant-based compound that gives many spices, such as turmeric, their bright yellow color. Some of the health benefits of turmeric are due to its active component: curcumin. Curcumin itself has poor bioavailability, meaning it has difficulty being absorbed by the body. However, recent studies have shown that when curcumin *is* absorbed, it tends to concentrate in the GI tract. Additionally, there is up to 2,000 percent increased absorption when curcumin is consumed with black pepper. These potent anti-inflammatory effects can benefit the lining of the digestive tract for those with LGS.

- **Fiber.** Dietary fiber is an important component of any healthy diet; it works in a similar way as probiotics to improve the microbiome. When fiber is fermented by the gut flora, it creates the short-chain amino acid butyrate.

- **L-Glutamine.** Glutamine is an amino acid that has been shown to improve the growth and survival of enterocytes, or intestinal cells. Research has also shown that glutamine can help regulate the function of the intestinal barrier during stress.

- **Probiotics.** I explained earlier how probiotics found in certain fermented foods and beverages can help treat LGS. These live microorganisms improve the microbiome of the gut. In a 14-week trial conducted in 2012, researchers studied the usefulness of a multi-strain probiotic supplement taken by participants after intense exercise. They found that zonulin, a marker of gut leakage, was significantly lower in the probiotic supplementation group.

- **Zinc.** Zinc is known for its ability to boost the immune system. A 2001 National Institutes of Health study found that zinc supplementation helped strengthen the gut lining in patients with Crohn's disease. This study and others suggest that zinc can modify the tight junctions of the intestinal lining, which helps reduce gut permeability. Zinc and copper levels need to be monitored by your physician if you take zinc for long periods of time.

It is essential to check with your doctor or pharmacist before taking any supplements and to ask about recommended doses for your individual condition. Make sure to follow their advice or the directions on the label. For best absorption, some dietary supplements should be taken with food; you may need to take others on an empty stomach. Fat-soluble vitamins should be taken with a meal containing some kind of fat to aid absorption.

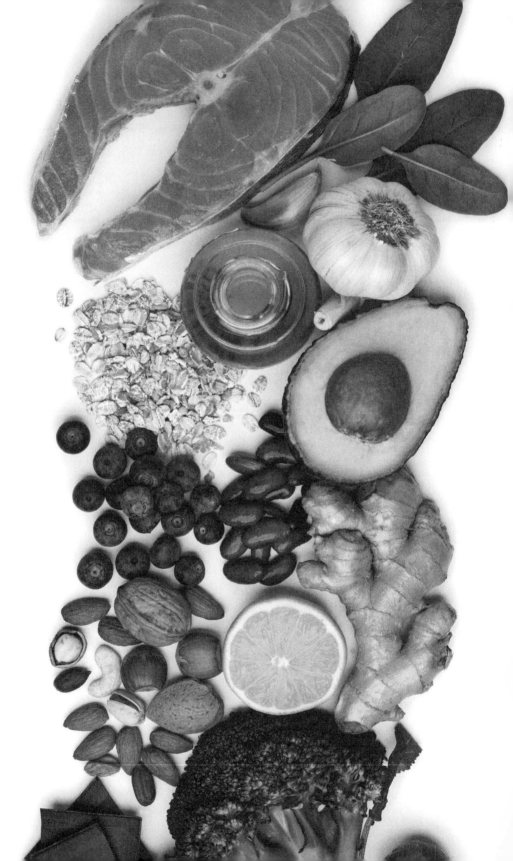

CHAPTER 10

Tips for Staying Motivated

Starting any new diet or change in lifestyle is a challenge, and even harder is staying the course. It's difficult to break old habits, especially if you've been eating the same way for years. Take heart (literally—the Heal Your Leaky Gut Diet is good for your heart as well as your stomach) and try the following tips if you're tempted to abandon ship:

1. **Take baby steps.** Taking small, measurable steps will help you achieve your larger goal. Writing your intentions down in your food diary also makes it feel more like a contract with yourself. Sample goals could be: "I will eat an additional serving of fruits and vegetables today," or "I will incorporate leafy greens into two of my meals each day," or "I will drink eight cups of water today." Research has shown that food diaries are successful for improving weight loss.

2. **Snack from the fridge.** Refrigerators keep things fresh, so most processed foods are not kept there. When craving an afternoon snack, stick with something from the fridge

instead of the cabinets or pantry, such as a sugar-free yogurt with fresh organic berries and honey or baby carrots with hummus.

3. **Mix it up.** Eating the same thing for lunch every day might be easier, but it can get boring. Look at the healthy recipes in this book and switch them up from week to week.

4. **Recruit your friends and family.** Like exercise buddies, teaming up with a like-minded pal or family member to join you on your journey to health will help inspire you and is much more fun than going it alone. And we can all benefit by eating a healthy diet!

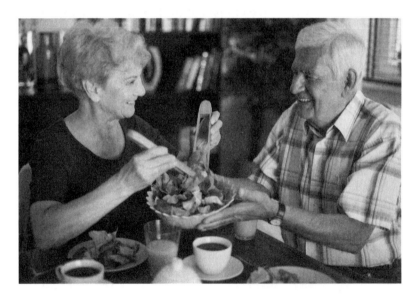

5. **Don't be hangry.** Many people get cranky when they're hungry. This is one reason it's a good idea to eat something every two to three hours. Doing this keeps

your metabolism active and prevents you from overeating (or eating the wrong foods) because you're ravenous and cranky.

6. **Keep nutritious foods handy.** Preparation is the key to eating healthy! Having fresh vegetables and fruits, lean protein, healthy fats, and smart carbs prepared in advance is a great way to stay on track. There's a reason fast food is so popular; people like to grab and go. Keep a week's worth of healthy goodie bags in the fridge that are ready to go for snacks and lunches.

7. **Avoid trigger foods.** Tempting foods that trigger you to overeat should not be in your kitchen. If ice cream is your weakness, for example, skip that particular frozen food section when shopping. If the tempting foods are already in your house because someone else bought them, try putting them away in a hard-to-reach cabinet or, better yet, get rid of them. Out of sight, out of mouth.

8. **Don't beat yourself up if you mess up.** We're all human, after all, so we are bound to falter every now and then. Don't let a setback keep you from your ultimate goal, which is healing your gut! Acknowledge that you slipped up and make sure that your next meal is a healthy one.

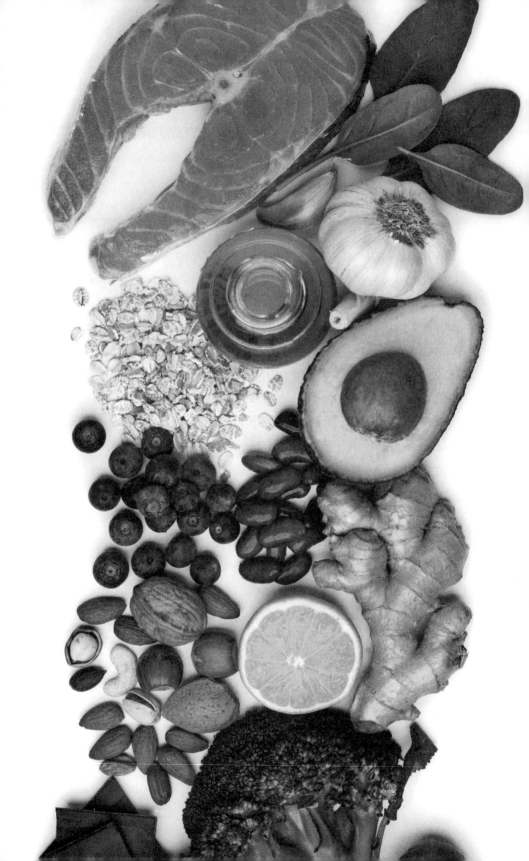

CHAPTER 11

Size Matters: Nine Tips for Portion Control

Unfortunately, many Americans "supersize" just about everything they eat and drink. I've found right-sizing to be one of the hardest habits for my patients to learn. The best place to start, I tell them, is to listen to your body. Your body will tell you when you are hungry; if you pay attention, you will know the difference between being truly (biologically) hungry and eating because you are stressed or bored.

Have you ever heard your stomach rumble or growl? This noise is caused by the squeezing of the GI tract to mix and propel food, gas, and fluids through the stomach and small intestines. Growling is associated with hunger because it is typically louder when the stomach and intestines are empty; the organs' contents don't muffle the noise. In later stages of hunger, you may feel light-headed, shaky, or even nauseated. These are all physical signs of hunger.

Similarly, when we are full, our bodies will tell us they are sated and satisfied. You might feel energized and clearheaded because you have the right amount of fuel for your brain to function properly. People with LGS often feel bloated after eating (especially when consuming the wrong kinds of foods), and keeping portions small is another helpful strategy for reducing bloating and intestinal distress. Here are some simple tips for eating and drinking a "just right" amount:

1. Use smaller plates and utensils.

Evidence suggests that the size of plates, spoons, and glasses can unconsciously influence how much food we eat and drink. Using large plates, for example, can make the food on them appear smaller, which often leads to overeating. In one notable study, nutrition experts served themselves 31 percent more ice cream when given larger bowls and 14.5 percent more when provided with larger serving spoons. Interestingly, most people who ate more due to large dishes were completely unaware of the change in portion size. The bottom line is switching your usual plates, bowls, or cutlery for smaller ones might reduce the amount of food you help yourself to and prevent you from overeating.

2. Use your plate as a portion guide.

Try using your plate or bowl as a portion-control guide. You can divide your plate into sections based on different food groups. This can help you determine the optimal ratio for a well-balanced meal. Here's a rough guide for lunch or dinner:

- Vegetables or salad: Half the plate
- High-quality protein: One quarter of the plate. This can be meat, poultry, fish, eggs, or beans.
- Complex carbs: One quarter of the plate. This can be whole grains or starchy vegetables.
- High-fat foods: Half a tablespoon of healthy oils or butter

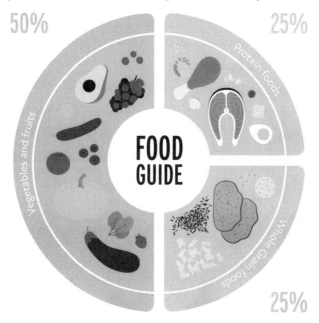

Because vegetables and salad are naturally high in fiber and other nutrients, filling up on these can help you avoid overeating. If you want extra guidance, some manufacturers sell portion-control plates (thedietplate.com).

3. Use your hands as a serving guide.

Another way to gauge appropriate portion size without any measuring tools is by simply using your hands. Our hands usually correspond to our body size, so bigger people, who require more food, typically have bigger hands. Here's another rough guide for each meal:

- High-protein foods: A palm-sized serving of meat, fish, poultry, or beans for women and two palm-sized portions for men
- Vegetables and salads: A fist-sized portion for women and two fist-sized portions for men
- High-carb foods: One cupped-hand portion for women and two for men—such as whole grains and starchy vegetables
- High-fat foods: One thumb-sized portion for women and two for men—such as butter, oils, and nuts

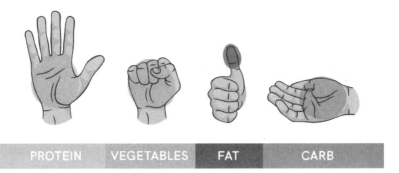

| PROTEIN | VEGETABLES | FAT | CARB |

4. Avoid All-You-Can-Eat Buffets

Stay away from all-you-can-eat buffets, where it's easy to overindulge and make several return trips to the table. If you do go to a buffet-style meal, use the dessert plate instead of the larger entree plate. Take your plate and move away from the table to engage in conversation with friends and family elsewhere. And remember the rules above when choosing how to fill your plate.

5. Start all meals with a glass of water.

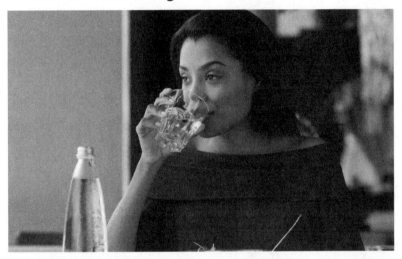

Remember the importance of drinking water? Drinking a glass of water up to 30 minutes before a meal will naturally aid portion control. Not only will you feel less hungry, but being well hydrated also helps you distinguish between hunger and thirst.

6. Never eat straight from the container.

We've all done it. When we're feeling tired or just plain lazy, we reach for a container of food from the fridge and dig in without using a bowl or plate. *Always* take the time to serve yourself a portion of whatever it is you are eating. Eating from jumbo-sized packages or large containers encourages overeating and lessens awareness of appropriate portion sizes. This is especially true for snacks, even if you're snacking on nuts. Rather than eating snacks from the original packaging, empty them into a small bowl to prevent eating more than you need.

7. Be aware of suitable serving size.

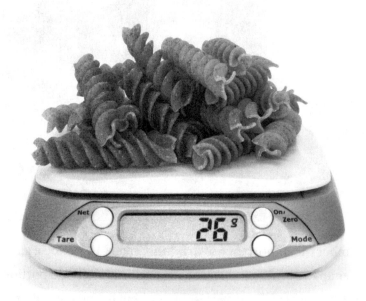

Research indicates that our own judgment is often faulty when it comes to appropriate portion size. Reading food labels is one way to increase awareness of how much we eat. (See page 147 on how to read labels.) Note the serving sizes on the package for commonly eaten foods to help you moderate your intake.

8. Use your food diary.

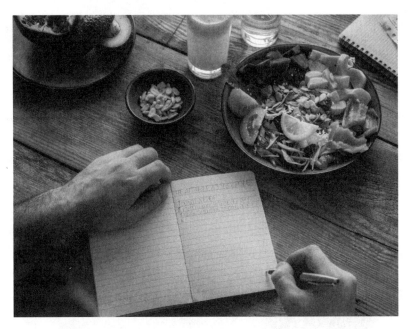

Studies show that people are often surprised by how much food they actually eat; this makes your food diary a helpful tool. The simple act of writing down what you eat and drink at each meal (and snack) increases your awareness of the type and amount of foods you're consuming.

9. Take your time.

The more you chew, the longer your meal will last and the less you will eat. As I mentioned earlier, most people do not chew their food properly, which can lead to poor digestion. I cannot emphasize enough the importance of taking the time to chew and savor your food.

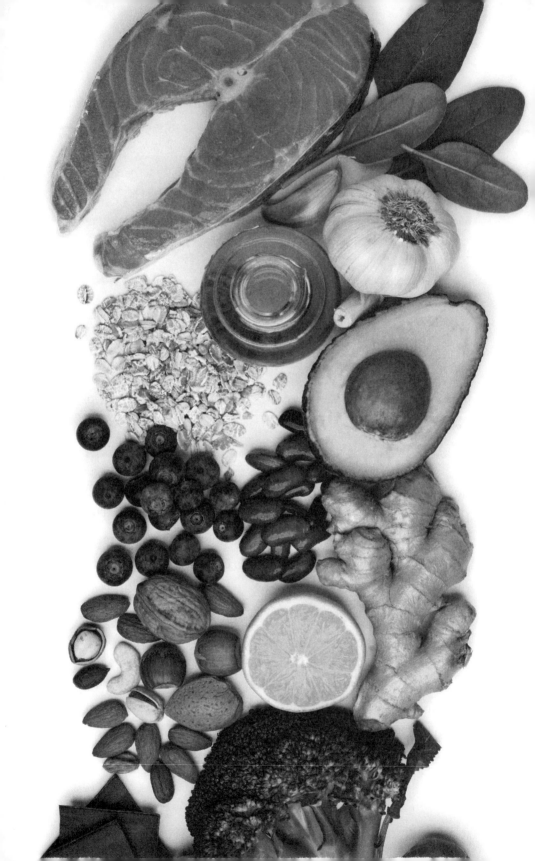

CHAPTER 12

How to Decipher Food Labels

In general, consumers are more health-conscious than ever. Because of this, many food manufacturers have begun to use misleading words or phrases on their labels to fool people into thinking that their highly processed products are actually healthy. Food-labeling regulations are complicated, making it even harder for average consumers to understand them. Get ready to learn how to read food labels so that you can differentiate between junk and truly healthy foods!

Look on the Back

One of the best tips I can give you is to ignore any claims on the front of the packaging. Front labels are essentially slick advertising promoting health claims. Many times, these claims have little or no basis in fact. Research shows that these claims on front labels make people believe a product is healthier than the exact same product without health claims on the label. Sadly, the practice of misleading consumers with false labeling is rampant. Examples include many high-sugar breakfast cereals

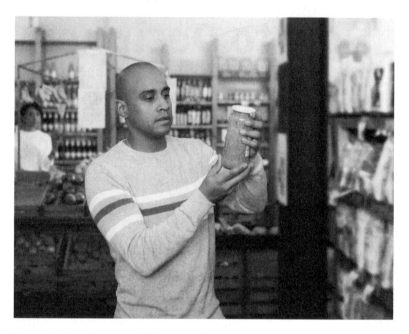

Read the Ingredients List

INGREDIENTS: ENRICHED FLOUR (WHEAT FLOUR, NIACIN, REDUCED IRON, THIAMIN MONONITRATE [VITAMIN B1], RIBOFLAVIN [VITAMIN B2], FOLIC ACID), CORN SYRUP, SUGAR, SOYBEAN AND PALM OIL (WITH TBHG FOR FRESHNESS), CORN SYRUP SOLIDS, DEXTROSE, HIGH FRUCTOSE CORN SYRUP, FRUCTOSE, GLYCERIN, CONTAINS 2% OR LESS OF COCOA (PROCESSED WITH ALKALI), POLYDEXTROSE, MODIFIED CORN STARCH, SALT, DRIED CREAM, CALCIUM CARBONATE, CORNSTARCH, LEAVING (BAKING SODA, SODIUM ACID PYROPHOSPHATE, MONO CALCIUM PHOSPHATE, CALCIUM SULFATE), DISTILLED MONOGLYCERIDES, HYDROGENATED PALM KERNEL OIL, SODIUM STEROL LACTYLATE, GELATIN, COLOR ADDED, SOY LECITHIN, DATE, NATURAL AND ARTIFICIAL FLAVOR, VANILLA EXTRACT, CARNAUBA WAX, XANTHAN GUM, VITAMIN A PALETTE, YELLOW #5 LAKE, RED #40 LAKE, CARAMEL COLOR, NIACIN AMIDE, BLUE #2 LAKE, REDUCED IRON, YELLOW #6 LAKE, PYRIDOXINE HYDROCHLORIDE (VITAMIN B6), RIBOFLAVIN (VITAMIN B2), THIAMIN HYDROCHLORIDE (VITAMIN B1), CITRIC ACID, FOLIC ACID, RED #40, YELLOW #5, YELLOW #6, BLUE #2, BLUE #1.

Carefully examine the ingredients list before you buy. Product ingredients are listed by quantity—from highest to lowest amount by weight. This means that the first ingredient is what the product contains most of. The first three ingredients on the label make up the largest part of what you're eating. If these ingredients include refined grains, any type of sugar, or hydrogenated oils, put the package back on the shelf. Instead, choose items that have whole foods listed as the top three ingredients. Also, if the ingredients list is longer than two to three lines and the words are unpronounceable, chances are the product is highly processed.

Reading ingredient lists gets easier with practice. Ask yourself these questions as you take a few minutes to read the ingredient list above.

- What are the first three ingredients?
- Does this product contain hydrogenated oils?
- Are there ingredients I can't pronounce?
- Is this a food that belongs in my shopping cart?

How did you do? Did you identify enriched flour, corn syrup, and sugar as the first three ingredients? That's a bad sign already. Further down, did you notice hydrogenated palm kernel oil? And what about sodium stearoyl lactylate? You probably figured out pretty quickly that this item needs to go back on the shelf!

*A Guide to Reading Nutrition Labels

1

Nutrition Facts

4 servings per container

Serving size   1 cup (180g)

2

Amount per serving

Calories   245

% Daily Value*

3

Total Fat 12g	**14%**
Saturated Fat 2g	**10%**
Trans Fat 0g	
Cholesterol 8mg	**3%**
Sodium 210mg	**9%**
Total Carbohydrate 34g	**12%**
Dietary Fiber 7g	**25%**
Total Sugars 5g	
Includes 4g Added Sugars	**8%**
Protein 11g	

4

Vitamin D 4mcg	20%
Calcium 210mg	16%
Iron 4mg	22%
Potassium 380mg	8%

5

*The % Daily Value (DV) tells you how much a nutrient in a serving of food contributes to a daily diet. 2,000 calories a day is used for general nutrition advice.

In the nutrition label above, look at how much sodium (salt) and sugar are in the product. For example, a can of Coke contains 39 grams of sugar! We should not be consuming any food product that has added refined sugar. Other things to look for on a food label include hydrogenated oils. Below are some tips for properly reading nutrition labels:

1. Read the serving information at the top.

This tells you the size of a single serving and the total number of servings per container or package.

2. Check the total calories per serving and container.

Pay attention to the calories per serving and how many calories you're consuming if you eat the whole package. If you eat two servings, you must double the calories and nutrients.

3. Check the nutrients.

Check key nutrients and understand what's on the list. Remember, not all fats are bad, and total sugars can include both natural and added sugars. Limit the amount of added sugars, saturated fat, and sodium (salt) you eat and avoid trans fat altogether. When choosing among different brands of similar products, always compare labels.

4. Look at the beneficial nutrients.

Make sure you get enough of the nutrients your body needs such as calcium, choline, dietary fiber, iron, magnesium, potassium, and vitamins A, C, D, and E.

5. Understand % Daily Value.

The % Daily Value (DV) tells you the percentage of each nutrient in a single serving in terms of the daily recommended amount. If you want to consume less of a nutrient (such as saturated fat or sodium), choose foods with a lower % DV (5 percent or less). If you want to consume more of a nutrient (such as fiber), choose foods with a higher % DV (20 percent or more).

*Source: The American Heart Association

What Label Terms Really Mean

Health claims on packaged food are often designed to grab your attention and to make you think that the product is healthy. Here are some of the most common terms—and what they *really* mean:

- **Light.** Light products are processed to reduce either calories or fat. Some products are simply watered down. Check carefully to see if anything has been added, such as sugar.
- **Multigrain.** Sounds healthy, right? What it actually means is that a product contains more than one type of grain. These are most likely refined grains—unless the product is marketed as whole grain.

- **Natural.** This is one of the most misleading terms. Arsenic is natural, but it sure isn't good for you! "Natural" simply indicates that at some point during the manufacturing process, the packager used a natural source like apples or rice.
- **No added sugar.** Some products, like orange juice, are naturally high in sugar. The fact that they don't have added sugar doesn't mean they're healthy. Plus, unhealthy sugar substitutes may have been added.
- **Low-calorie.** Low-calorie products have to have one-third fewer calories than the brand's original product. One brand's low-calorie version may have the same number of calories as another brand's original.
- **Low-fat.** This label usually means that the fat has been reduced; however, more sugar was likely added to make the product taste better. If a product says it's low-fat, read the ingredients list with a skeptical eye.
- **Low-carb.** The popular keto and paleo diets are extremely low in carbs. Be aware, however, that processed foods labeled as low-carb can still be unhealthy foods, similar to processed low-fat foods.
- **Made with whole grains.** Despite this healthy-sounding phrase, the product may contain few whole grains. Remember the order of ingredients? Check the ingredient list—if whole grains aren't in the first three ingredients, the amount is negligible.

- **Fortified or enriched.** This means that some nutrients have been added to the product. Vitamin D is often added to milk, for example. Just because something is fortified doesn't make it good for you.
- **Gluten-free.** As I mentioned in Chapter 2, many gluten-free foods are highly processed and loaded with unhealthy fats and sugar.
- **Fruit-flavored.** A "flavor" can be manufactured in a lab with chemicals to taste and smell like the real thing. Some processed strawberry yogurts may not contain any fruit.
- **Cage-free.** The USDA states that eggs labeled as cage-free "must be produced by hens housed in a building, room, or enclosed area that allows for unlimited access to food, water, and provides the freedom to roam within the area during the laying cycle." In other words, *the hens are still enclosed.*
- **Free-range.** Eggs labeled as free-range must be produced by hens that have unlimited access to food and water and access to the outdoors during their egg-laying cycle. Free-range eggs are a better food source compared to conventionally produced eggs.
- **Pasture-raised.** This term refers to an animal raised for food, and you'll find it as a label on meat, dairy, and eggs. Research has found that one pasture-raised egg contains twice as much omega-3 fat, three times more vitamin D, four times more vitamin E, and seven times more beta-carotene than an egg from a hen raised on traditional

feed. There are similar nutritional benefits to meat from grass-fed cattle. Another thing to look for are the words "certified humane" on the package.

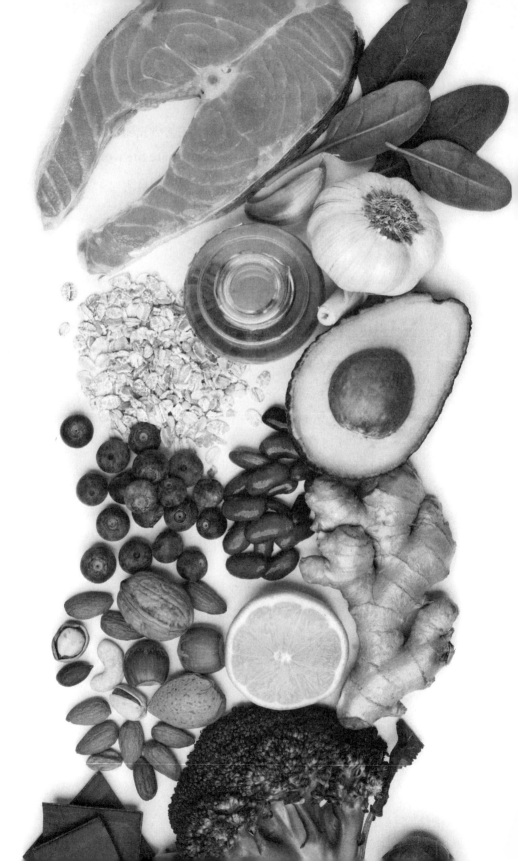

CHAPTER 13

Where to Get Specialty Foods

The good news is that gluten-free and dairy-free products are now available at many grocery and health food stores. If you prefer to shop online, here are some companies that will deliver the healthy goods directly to your home:

Thrive Market (thrivemarket.com)
This site sells thousands of curated foods, from organic pantry staples to supplements and sustainable meat for 70+ different diets. Shop à la carte or get a monthly membership.

Imperfect Foods (try.imperfectfoods.com)
Help prevent food waste and support local farmers by ordering your own customized box of organic produce that would otherwise be discarded. These items may be "ugly" looking, but they are nutritionally perfect. You get charged only when the food arrives.

ButcherBox (butcherbox.com)

ButcherBox devotes itself to selling high-quality, humanely raised meat. Each month, they deliver 100 percent grass-fed beef, humanely raised pork, and free-range organic chicken straight to your door. They partner only with companies and farmers who are dedicated to producing high-quality protein for families across the country.

Farmbox Direct (try.farmboxdirect.com)

This fresh produce delivery service partners with a network of farms to deliver healthy, organic fruits and vegetables to your table. Choose your box size and customize it to your liking. You get up to five seasonal veggies or fruits in each weekly or biweekly order.

Shop at Your Local Farmers Market

The best way to support small farms is to shop at your local farmers market. Nearly every town or city has one, so find out where they are located near you. Search this national database of farmers markets at www.localharvest.org/.

Community Supported Agriculture (CSA)

You might want to consider joining a CSA, which allows you to buy directly from farms. Being part of a CSA or Farm Share program is different from shopping at your local grocery store. Members pre-pay for a share of the upcoming season's harvest and receive fresh, clean, and nutritious produce straight from the farm to your table. You can find information on CSAs on localharvest.org.

ACKNOWLEDGMENTS

I gratefully acknowledge the help I have received from Jodie Gould in putting this book together. Jodie was instrumental in creating this book.

Thank you to Mary Glenn at Humanix Books for your encouragement and support.

Finally, thanks to Chris Ruddy and Newsmax for all the support and allowing me to have an unfiltered voice.

I would also like to thank my patients. Your search for safe and effective natural treatments is the driving force behind holistic medicine. You have accompanied me down this path, and I appreciate each and every one of you.